The Publisher would like to thank Mrs Wendy
Thomson and her sister Mrs Daphnie Harris for
bringing to his attention the possible benefits of
Magnet Therapy together with the assistance and help
which assisted in the publication of this book

Published in 2002 by Caxton Editions
20 Bloomsbury Street
London WC1B 3JH
a member of the Caxton Publishing Group

Designed and produced for Caxton Editions
by Open Door Limited
Rutland, United Kingdom

Editing: Mary Morton
Typesetting: Jane Booth
Digital imagery © copyright 2002 PhotoDisc Inc.

Title: Magnetic Therapy
ISBN: 1 84067 390 7

IMPORTANT NOTICE
This book is not intended to be a substitute for medical
advice or treatment. Any person with a condition requiring
medical attention should consult a qualified medical
practitioner or therapist.

MAGNETIC THERAPY

GLORIA VEGARI

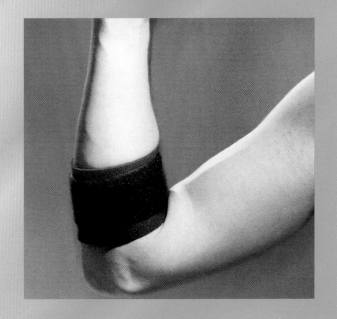

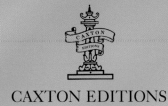

CAXTON EDITIONS

CONTENTS

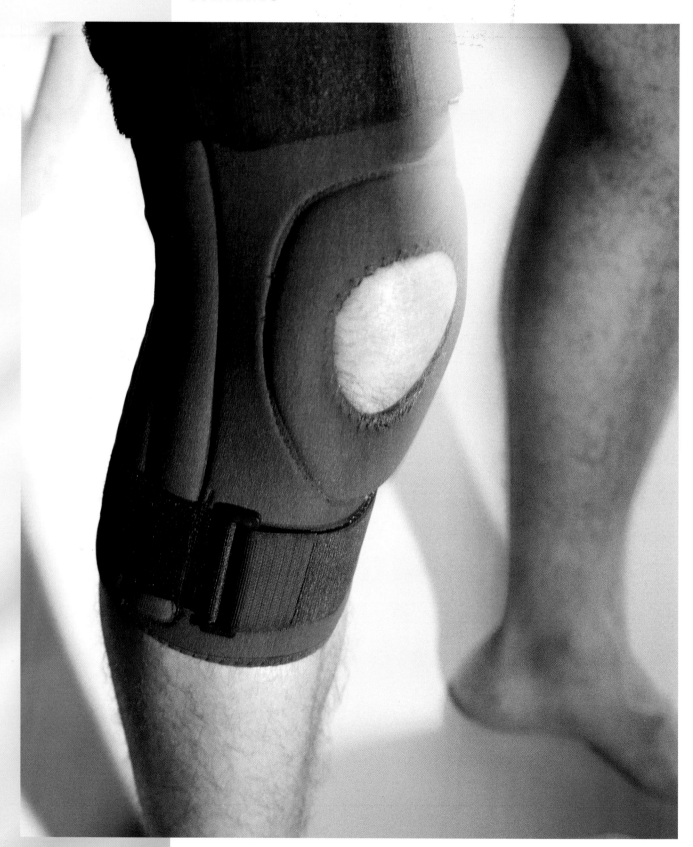

CONTENTS

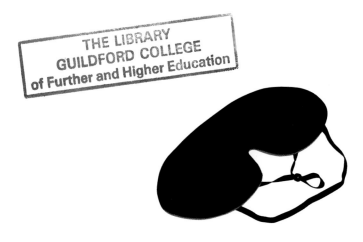

PREFACE

MAGNET THERAPY
By Gloria Vergari MCMA

Gloria Vergari is one of the first magnet therapists in England to be accredited by the Complementary Medical Association (CMA) Prior to that she studied magnet therapy in America under Jim Souder, one of the leaders in the technology of biomagnetic therapy in the USA.

She has devoted the last five years to pushing forward this new frontier in healthcare. In that period she has worked with over 3,000 patients.

Below: 'magnets are not magic. Their function is very simple.'

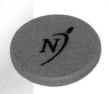

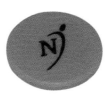

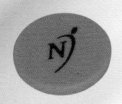

MAGNET THERAPY IS NOT:
- A miracle or the answer to everything.
- To be used without a diagnosis.
- To be used by persons using a pacemaker, defibrillator, insulin pump or other electro-insulin device.
- To be used by pregnant women.

MAGNET THERAPY IS:
- Doctor-recommended.
- Clinically tested.
- Safe and effective.
- Re-usable.
- A non-invasive drug-free therapy.
- Affordable.

According to **Dr Ken Wianko**, a prominent American physician: 'Magnets are not magic. Their function is very simple. Magnotherapy helps the body regain its self-healing balance naturally, because each organ and cell in the body is influenced by magnetic fields. Cell regulation, tissue function and life itself are controlled by electromagnetic currents.'

'I honestly believe that simply wearing a modern magnet is one of the easiest ways we can enhance our well-being.'
Gloria Vergari MCMA in The Handbook to Understanding Magnet Therapy

INTRODUCTION

Before I take you through the basics of magnet therapy (or magnotherapy) and how it works, let me clear up some of the questions I am most frequently asked.

Why have I only recently heard of it?

Where did it come from?

Is it safe?

How should I use it?

Stay with me – this will be a fascinating journey and one that could change the way you approach looking after your family's healthcare.

Nowadays the possibility of our living to be 80 or 90 is practically taken for granted, and when we or our loved ones don't make it we almost feel slighted. However, with this long lease on life comes the realisation that the NHS cannot and will not be there for every ache and pain – which means we will have to become familiar with ways of healing and maintaining our own bodies. The general trend is to look for more natural ways of doing so. Over the last few years, people in the UK and throughout the world have opened up to complementary and alternative medicine, actively searching for non–intrusive, drug-free and, above all, safe methods that are known to work. We are entering a new era in self-managed health care, when 'soft' medical alternatives are increasingly preferred over drugs and surgery whenever possible.

Magnotherapy is all of the above, and more. In this book we will attempt to explain how magnets effect changes, and answer some of your questions, simply and frankly.

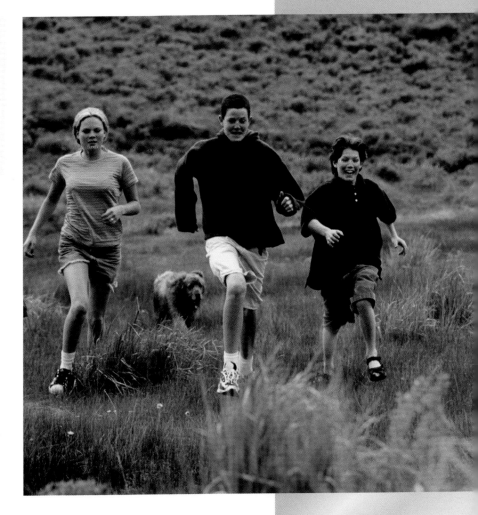

Above: the possibility of our living to be 80 or 90 is practically taken for granted, especially when we are young and full of energy.

THE IMPORTANCE OF MAGNETIC FIELDS AND ENERGY

The universe, as Douglas Adams says in *The Hitchhiker's Guide to The Galaxy*, '... is big, it's very big'.

It is; think of all those planets, moons and stars out there, just hanging around in space. What is it that keeps them in their own particular place and not crashing into each other? Yes, you have it – gravity and magnetic fields continually pulling and opposing and holding the planets, moons and stars in their appointed place or orbit.

The Earth is, in fact, a giant magnet. Courtesy of Einstein and other physicists we now have terms for the four forces which give and maintain order on our planet and in the universe: the weak nuclear force, the strong nuclear force, gravity, and the electromagnetic.

The Earth, mankind, animals, cells, atoms – life itself – are exposed to and charged with terrestrial magnetic fields. Every cell in our body has some energy or force flowing through it. To quote Shakespeare, not only are we 'such stuff that dreams are made of', but we are also made up from the dust of ancient stars. Isn't that a lovely thought to hang onto as we are fighting the rush-hour crowds?

In that dust are tiny magnetic particles. When we are attracted to someone and say they have a magnetic personality or that there is some 'chemistry' happening, we are right – each of us gives off greater or lesser energies at slightly different strengths. A few people with a natural high output can become healers. The rest of us can now do the same to our own bodies by using therapeutic magnets.

Below: the Earth is in fact a giant magnet.

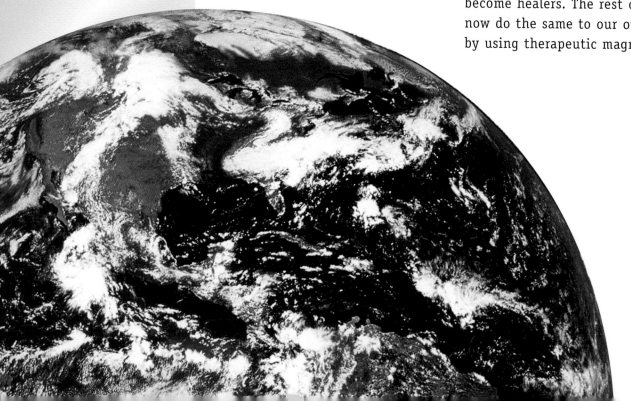

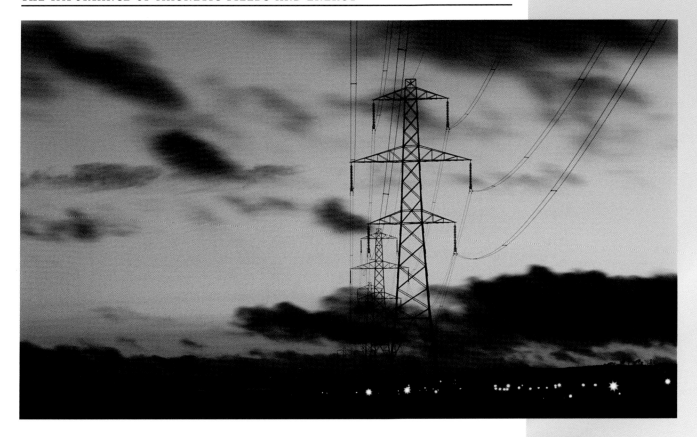

Remember the old cliché 'opposites attract'. The fact is that opposites are dynamic, creating change, pushing us ever forward. Positive and negative, yin and yang, hot and cold, dark and light, the moon, sun and earth are working towards our well-being. This energy field we were born into is vital for our health.

But these days we are receiving less of the natural magnetic field we used to get from the planet. Modern life 'insulates' us. We no longer walk barefoot on the earth. Most of us in the Western world live and work in concrete buildings and we travel everywhere in metal cars, trains or planes. This, combined with the electricity we surround ourselves with daily, bombards our bodies, causing stress to our cells. Radio waves, used to transmit television and radio, microwaves from satellites, electric fields from overhead cables and even our own home lighting and power have depleted a significant amount of our own natural energy source. Just how is yet to be determined, but there is a lot of research going on into the causes and triggers for such 'modern' diseases as chronic fatigue syndrome (CFS), magnetic deficiency syndrome (MDS), multiple sclerosis (MS) and most notably myalgic encephalitis (ME) .

Above: electric fields from overhead cables and even our own home lighting have depleted our own natural energy.

Roger Coghill, one of Britain's most noted researchers in the area of energy fields and medicine, tells us how, when a metal object is placed in an electric field, that field will be conducted to each part of the object.

In one case study he noted how a patient suffering from ME slept in a brass bed. At the back of the metal headboard was a double electric socket feeding two bedside lamps and a clock/radio, which were naturally kept switched on, merrily transmitting all through the night. Roger immediately re-positioned the bed, and the patient shortly saw improvements in her health and strength.

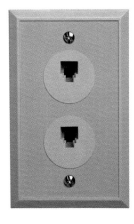

We have been brought up taking the benefits of electricity for granted; they are all too apparent in our daily lives. None of us would dream of turning back the clock and living without electric power, but it may have taken a toll on our system, and we may have to become somewhat clearer and more discerning in how we use it.

According to scientists the Earth has lost over 5 per cent of its magnetic field in the last century, and adding the two things together you can see that we may be functioning slightly under par – our 'batteries' may have had the edge taken off them.

Strangely enough, two places on Earth are said to have a higher magnetic reading than others – one is **Sedona in Arizona**, the other is **Lourdes in France**.

Right: we have been brought up taking the benefits of electricity for granted.

Below: none of us would dream of turning back the clock and living without electric power, but it may have taken a toll on our system.

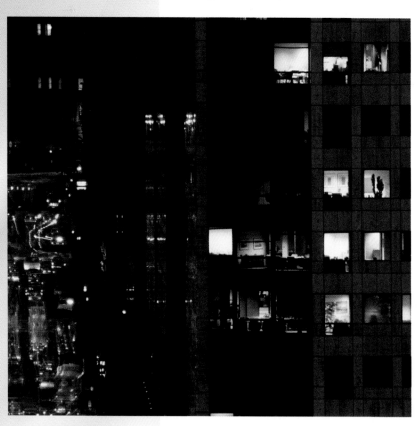

A SHORT HISTORY OF MEDICINE

2000BC	*Here, eat this root.*
1000AD	*That root is heathen. Here, say this prayer.*
1850AD	*That prayer is superstition. Here, drink this potion.*
1940AD	*That potion is snake oil. Here, swallow this pill.*
1985AD	*That pill is ineffective. Here, take this antibiotic.*
2000AD	*That antibiotic is artificial. Here, eat this root.*

Below: yin and yang – the understanding derived from two opposite influences that balance each other out.

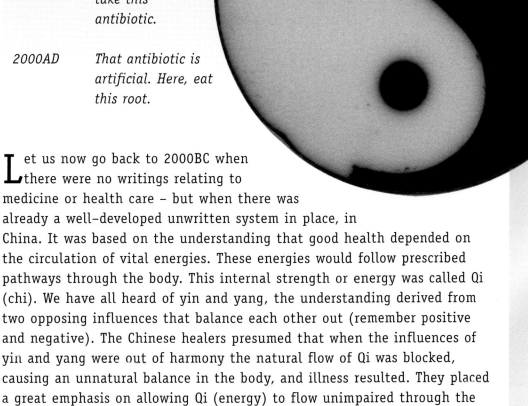

Let us now go back to 2000BC when there were no writings relating to medicine or health care – but when there was already a well-developed unwritten system in place, in China. It was based on the understanding that good health depended on the circulation of vital energies. These energies would follow prescribed pathways through the body. This internal strength or energy was called Qi (chi). We have all heard of yin and yang, the understanding derived from two opposing influences that balance each other out (remember positive and negative). The Chinese healers presumed that when the influences of yin and yang were out of harmony the natural flow of Qi was blocked, causing an unnatural balance in the body, and illness resulted. They placed a great emphasis on allowing Qi (energy) to flow unimpaired through the body.

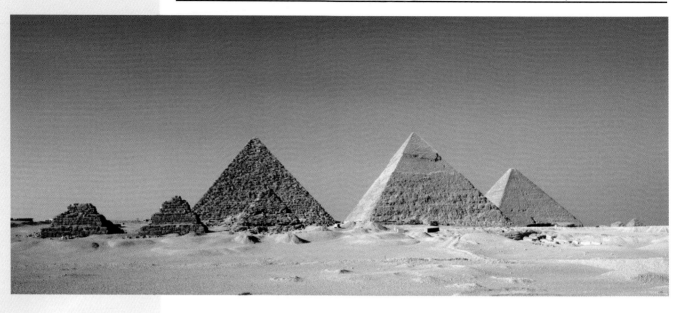

Above: Egyptian physicians used lodestones (magnets) for a variety of conditions. Queen Cleopatra herself wore a small magnet in an amulet on her forehead to preserve her youth.

It was in this period that the first work on healing was written; it was called *The Emperor's Book of Internal Medicine*. This book described how imbalances could be corrected by what we now know to be acupuncture – and the use of magnetic stones. The Chinese author went on to explain how key points in the body related to different organs and energy lines.

Egyptian physicians used lodestones (magnets) for a variety of conditions. Queen Cleopatra herself wore a small magnet in an amulet on her forehead to preserve her youth. We know today how right she was, but how did she know this? At the back of the forehead lies the pineal gland; this is quite small (about the size if a pine nut). The pineal is home to melatonin, which is secreted by the gland at night. Melatonin is a powerful

antioxidant and is now being hailed as the 'youth hormone' due to its anti–ageing capacities. So Cleo was right on the nose – or, rather, forehead!

Today, instead of hanging an amulet on our forehead, we can simply sleep on a magnetic pillow pad to achieve the same result – it is like having an eight-hour beauty treatment while we sleep. Melatonin in pill form has become very popular as a sleep aid and is used widely for jetlag and regulating sleep patterns. Again, sleeping on a magnetic pad will encourage the pineal gland to secrete melatonin naturally and thus secure the same result as the pill.

Thales, a seventh-century BC Greek philosopher, said, 'All things are full of gods'. He made this remark when noting that if amber, which is a fossilised tree resin, was rubbed with wool, it would pick up light objects such as straw or feathers. Somehow it 'attracted' them. The Greeks were also the first people to understand the properties of magnetite and how this grey stone could attract nails and other items made of iron. Thales thought that magnetite (lodestone) 'has soul because it attracts iron'. The Greeks saw these things as magic from the gods. They saw the effects these special stones could have in healing and worked with them, believing the gods used them to intervene and help mankind.

We can skip through the Dark Ages, acknowledge the part played by Paracelsus (1493–1541) in furthering our understanding of magnets, note the part he foresaw them playing in healing both in humans and animals and come to the time of Elizabeth I. It is widely reported that her personal physician Dr William Gilbert (1540–1600) would treat strangulated hernia (twisted hernia) by using iron filings. Dr Gilbert would have

the filings baked into a cake, then feed the cakes to his patient, and wait for them to be digested. By placing a lodestone over the lower stomach area he would untwist the hernia. How about that for non-invasive surgery? Dr Gilbert also believed that whatever strange force existed in magnets, it was the key to life.

Just look at Michelangelo's painting on the ceiling of the Sistine Chapel – it shows Adam being animated by God with what appears to be the 'spark of life'.

Below: a seventh-century BC Greek philosopher, said, 'All things are full of gods'. He made this remark when noting that if amber, which is a fossilised tree resin, was rubbed with wool, it would pick up light objects such as straw or feathers.

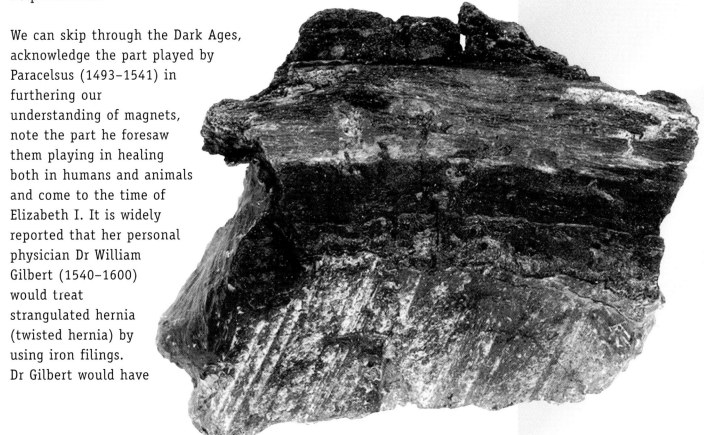

In the 18th and 19th centuries many noted scientists and physicians experimented with magnetic fields and electricity. Their knowledge and the materials they had were pretty crude, but they had valiant stabs at understanding principles which we today are becoming more and more aware of – that energy medicine could point the way to the next generation of healing.

One of these young academic doctors was Franz Mesmer. Today he is somewhat ridiculed as the 'quack' who used to hypnotise his patients, hence, the word 'mesmerise'. Mesmer was, in fact, a brilliant young man who studied mathematics, the law and medicine. His doctoral thesis dealt with the effects of gravitational fields and cycles on human health. Over the years he practised medicine, using magnets and patients from all over Europe flocked to him. His popularity grew by word of mouth and he became one of the most successful and controversial men in France. The medical community was, as always, conservative and distrustful. They thought he was a fraud and all the cures he achieved were due to his powers of suggestion. In other words, he 'mesmerised' his patients.

If only Mesmer were alive today, to see the modern magnets and magnetic materials being used in magnet therapy, he would be completely vindicated and respected for the visionary and scientist he was.

Today Tibetan monks still place large lodestones around the head for clarity of thought to improve the concentration and learning capacity of young monks in training.

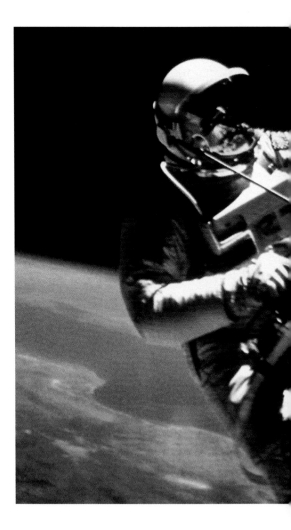

MODERN (OR THERAPEUTIC) MAGNETS

It is said that we owe the development of modern 'medical' magnets to the space industry. Certainly the industry played a major part in developing the materials we now use in magnet and biomagnetic therapies. It was also responsible for introducing a wider audience to the vital role the Earth's magnetic field has on the human body.

When man first ventured into space in the 1960s, we understood the need to provide him with a safe, reliable space craft, the astronaut was given a life-supporting suit and went through a thorough training programme to withstand the mental and physical challenges we understood he would encounter. He was then sent off into the unknown and the space agencies made sure the back-up on Earth was of the highest calibre.

We know just how successful both the Americans and Russians were in this enterprise. We were amazed and delighted to see the astronauts return from their pioneering endeavours, tired but safe and smiling. After the very first space flights, the astronauts needed to be placed in isolation for several weeks upon their return. It was discovered from the constant monitoring from Earth during their flights that when they were in space the men were losing bone density and calcium and their immune systems became depleted. During the quarantine period that followed a flight, it became clear that the physio-logical changes that occurred were partly a result of man leaving the Earth's magnetic field. As I mentioned before this magnetic energy field is something we are born into, humans as a species evolve in it, and without it our bodies suffer. We lose the energy (Qi) to produce the normal level of bodily function we and other living things need to survive.

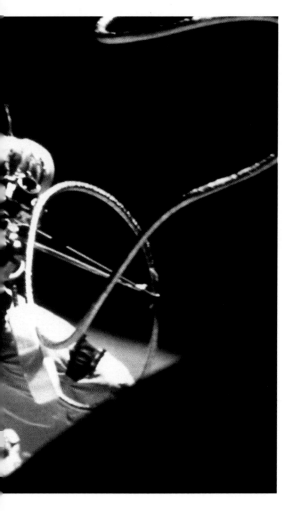

Left: the space industry has played a major part in the development of modern 'medical' magnets.

What to do?

Whether it was the Russians or the Americans who first came to understand the nature of the problem is not quite certain, but it was decided to place large magnetic blocks inside each spacecraft. This did begin to alleviate the problems. However, the increased load affected the fuel efficiency of the crafts on take-off. Therefore another solution had to be found.

The space agencies approached outside businesses and asked for them to develop extremely high-powered magnets that were lightweight. This they did, very successfully. For example, a magnet holding a note on your fridge door is 100 gauss – and a magnet we now use in health care can be the same size and weight and hold a magnetic strength of – **12,300 gauss**.

They came up with several of the materials that we now use and I will explain them in the next chapter.

Today, when astronauts go into space they wear suits lined with flexible magnetic materials and the spacecraft has a magnetic lining. Now when they return from a flight, whether it has been two days or two months, they go straight from the craft and into a press conference. This is the difference maintaining a magnetic balance can make to the human body.

THE WORLDWIDE USE OF MAGNETS:

In countries that are not dominated by a drug culture, as we in the West are, magnetic therapy is very often the first way of tackling soft-tissue damage. Countries such as Japan, Russia and China use it continually.

Over the last few years countries such as Germany and most recently the USA are fast catching on to the benefits of this exceptional therapy.

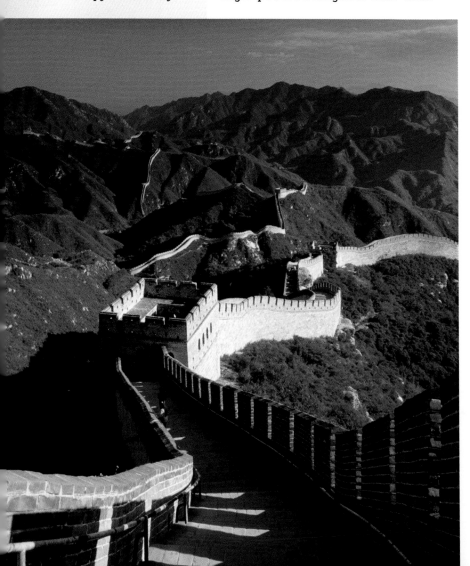

Below: countries that are not dominated by a drug culture such as Japan, Russia and China use magnet therapy continually.

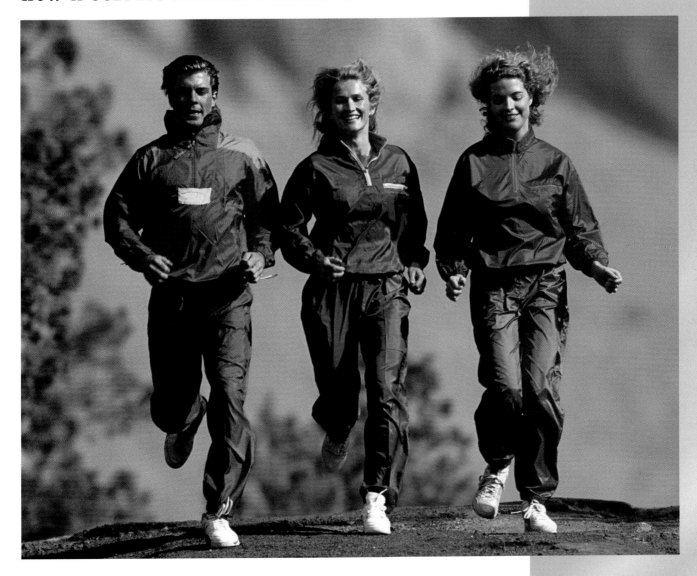

Above: whilst jogging one evening, my knee gave out.

Thirty years ago I had a serious knee accident when, as a professional dancer, I fell during one of the more active scenes in *West Side Story*. I heard several bones crack yet managed to hobble off stage and get myself down to Charing Cross Hospital in London. Over the next few months I was cut, stitched and screwed back together. The bones finally mended, but the ligaments remained a problem.

Though I can get by in most activities and sports, my knee does not like concrete and, whilst jogging one evening in 1997 with friends in North Carolina, my knee gave out and I was in severe pain. I asked them to book an appointment the following day with a local physiotherapist. This injury was an 'old friend' and I knew I needed a few sessions of ultra-sound and some anti-inflammatory pills.

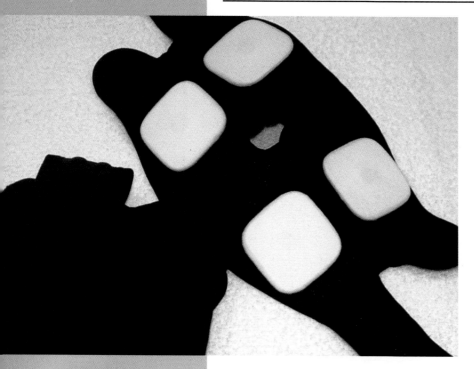

Above: one of my pals handed me a knee wrap which had magnets in it.

One of my pals handed me a knee wrap and said, 'here try this until morning'. I asked what it was and when he told me it had magnets in it, I politely told him to get lost. Some new gimmick from America, I thought! He insisted I try it. I refused and so on until he wore me down and I agreed to keep it on until I saw the physio in the morning. The following morning I got up, took the wrap off to shower, and low and behold there was not a trace of inflammation in my leg. I gingerly handed it back to my friend and said thanks. I thought it was interesting, but would not believe the wrap had anything to do with it – I wanted to believe my knee had just spontaneously healed. In 30 years it had never done so before, but a magnet? Well, really! I dismissed the idea.

Two weeks later, whilst moving a table in their house, I tore a muscle in my shoulder. Obviously somewhere in my deep unconscious I had remembered the magnets, because I asked them if I could stick the knee wrap over my shoulder. They laughed, said I would look like Quasimodo, and took me to the magnet therapist they had bought the knee wrap from. After a brief consultation, I was told that all I needed for my torn muscle was a powerful neodymium magnet. It was the size and weight of a 2p coin, but had the horsepower of a tank (12,300 gauss). Donna, the therapist, simply attached it to the most painful spot using medical tape. Within 24 hours the pain was gone and I had full mobility in arm and shoulder.

This now had my full attention. Over the years I had suffered enough injuries dancing, teaching aerobics and skiing to know something was happening inside my body. I went back to the therapist and she spent time with me, explaining the basics of what happened when a magnetic field is applied to the body, and how this new method of healing was sweeping the USA. In spite of the drug companies trying to discredit it, the public knew it worked and millions of Americans were now using it.

I was becoming extremely interested in the science behind it and Donna advised me to go down to Raleigh, North Carolina, and talk to one of the leaders in the research and development of biomagnetics, **Jim Souder**. Jim is respected throughout the community as a man of great integrity and a true innovator in the field. I went to Jim's clinic and stayed in his house and studied with him and his wife Judi for several months. They opened up a new world to me and, on my return to England I decided to spend time testing magnets. I did so, on friends, family and neighbours and their animals.

I was staggered by the results. Five years on and 3,000 patients later, I still find it hard to believe something this small and simple can actually be so effective in dealing with a wide variety of conditions – usually conditions that doctors have given up on.

At this point I decided to throw caution and money to the wind and give up a career that had been very lucrative to me for 17 years in order to pursue this subject. I took a deep breath and began to practise and study everything I came across concerning the therapeutic use of magnets.

I was not happy that in England there appeared to be no standards in place for therapists and, by pure chance, I met Valerie Dargonne, a young woman who had been independently studying this field for years. We both had similar intentions and aims for the future of magnets in the UK. We both wanted to get this therapy taken seriously by medical and professional healthcare practitioners. To date there are no legal requirements to establish oneself as a magnet therapist. Any multi-level marketer can sell magnets without truly understanding how and when to use them. Valerie and I wanted to establish some sort of standard of practice and, with this in mind, we decided a comprehensive training programme needed to be established here. Over several months Valerie developed our course, and to date we have trained and accredited 20 therapists, four doctors, three dentists, with more coming on board daily. We are the only school of magnet therapy to be accredited by The Complementary Medical Association in Britain.

I hope I can now share with you this simple therapy.

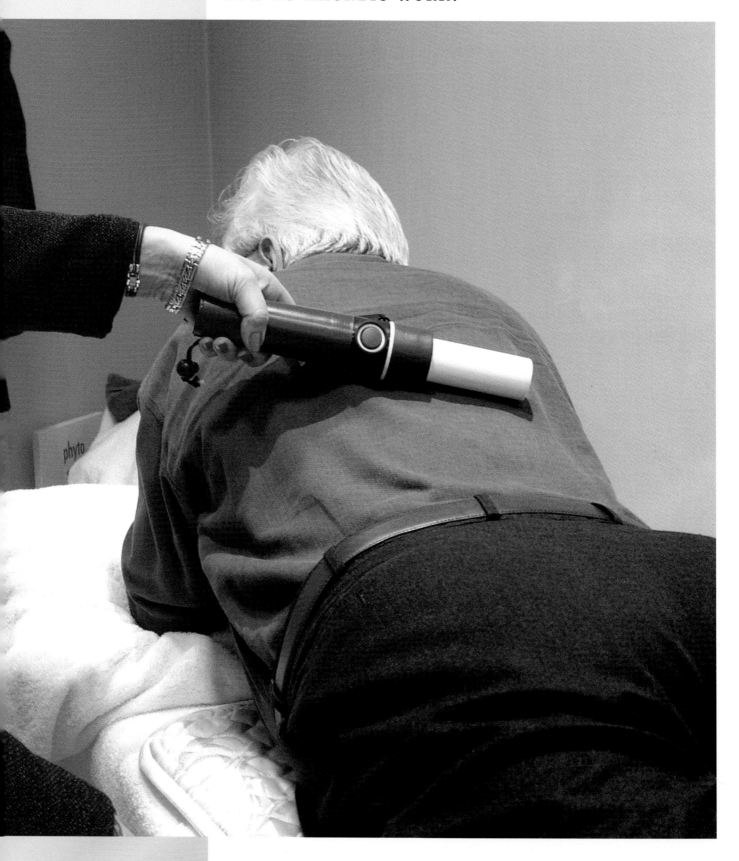

There is still much research and debate about how magnets work. Different theories have been put forward by manufacturers of magnetic products. I will summarise the largely accepted views held by doctors and researchers.

When a magnet is applied to the body, muscles and soft tissue lengthen and relax, waves pass through the tissue and secondary currents are induced. When those currents clash with magnetic waves they produce impacting heat on electrons in the body cells. These impacting heats are very effective in the reduction of muscle swelling and pain. Movement of haemoglobin in the blood vessels is accelerated – this has been observed in both thermographic and nuclear medicine studies – while calcium, cholesterol and lactic acid deposits in the blood are decreased. The fatigued blood is cleansed and circulation is increased. There is also significant evidence of a pain- blocking mechanism in nerve fibres themselves when subjected to magnetic fields. Researchers have been able to shift the resting potential (thereby raising the required stimulus to pain) of nerve cells in the laboratory by 25 per cent using the Norso Dynamag technology. High-strength magnets can cause anaesthesia, in the tissue, through a principal in physics called the Hall Effect, a thermal impact that occurs within the cell which can affect nerve signals.

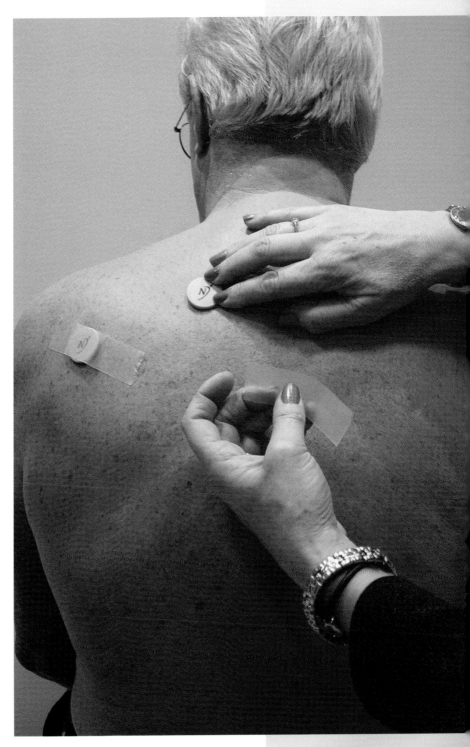

Below: when a magnet is applied to the body muscles and soft tissue lengthen and relax.

What does this all mean in lay terms?

Two vital things occur when a magnet is placed on the skin.

The soft tissue will lengthen and help to relax a muscle or ligament that is damaged/traumatised. It will work in an area and depth directly proportionate to the type and strength of magnet used. Presuming you have one of the better magnets – I will give you the guidelines in the following chapter– you should be able to effect a change to a radius of between 3–5 inches around any one magnet and to a similar depth.

As the tissue relaxes blood flow that has been blocked from entering the damaged site is allowed in and increased. We can see this by thermal imaging.

Normally an injured site, whether arthritis, torn muscles or another condition, will be surrounded by inflammation. This can consist of lactic acids, calcium and other deposits – basically the site is 'hot' with acidity. The increase in blood flow brings with it increased alkalinity. Acidity hates to be in an alkaline environment and this is where the body starts to generate its own healing. Magnets merely encourage it in a truly dramatic way.

So, we have relaxed the tissue and, with increased blood flow, we have started to detoxify the area. Next, the thermal impact I mentioned occurs inside the cell. As the blood in our body continuously circulates it periodically comes close to the magnet placed on the skin above. The ions in the blood become agitated and are attracted to the magnet, atomic particles begin to spin inside the cell, they go into the Hall Effect and in doing so get 'switched on'.

This 'switching on' means the body kicks in with its own beta-endorphin (pain-relieving) system.

Below: a wristband or sufficiently strong bracelet is fine if you have hand or wrist pain.

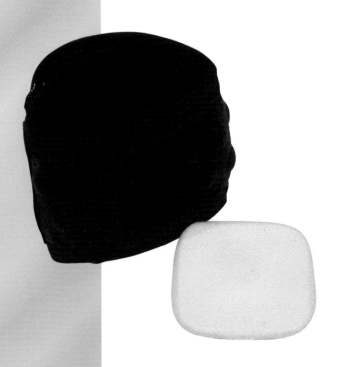

So to recap, we have:
1. *lengthened and relaxed tissue;*
2. *begun the process of flushing out debris and inflammation from the site;*
3. *kicked in the body's own pain-relieving system.*

These are the key points a user of magnetic products must understand if you wish to treat yourself and your family successfully. If you understand that the product works where it is placed, you will not fall into the trap of buying a wristband to help with pain in your knee.

If a magnet is going to work for you, it can happen within hours when quality magnets are placed over the damaged area. Normally we expect to see improvements within 1 –7 days, **when you are directly treating the site of pain**.

A wristband or sufficiently strong bracelet is fine if you have hand or wrist pain, or if you want to maximise your general health and detox you body. You will keep it there, as it is easy to wear there. But there is little point in relaxing and promoting blood flow to your wrist if your problem is your lower back!

Wearing a magnet anywhere on the body will still have the same detoxifying effect on the blood, after a period of time. As I

mentioned before, the agitation within the circulating cells releases the debris that clings to the walls of the cell. One thing you must remember when you use magnet therapy is to drink at least 4–5 glasses of water a day. You need to flush out of your system the toxins the magnets are releasing. Coffee, tea (whether herbal or not) and fruit juice are just not the same as water. The liver reads them as food.

We are 75 per cent water and we need to replenish the cells. It does not matter whether it is spring, mineral or tap – just WATER.

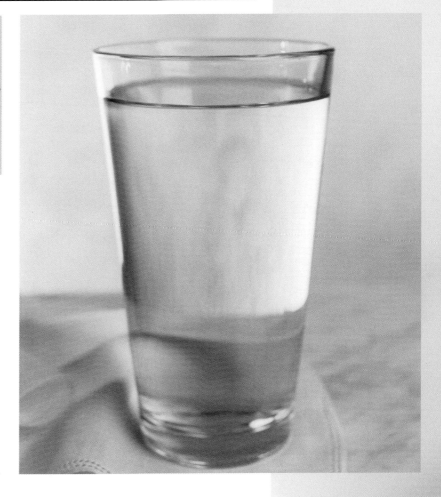

Above: when you use magnet therapy it is important to drink at least 4–5 glasses of water a day.

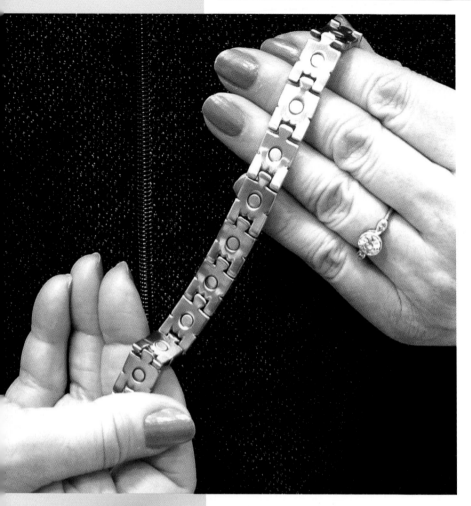

Above: choose a 'north-pole' bracelet and make sure it is sufficiently strong to affect changes. This bracelet has magnets embedded all the way along the underside

MAIN BENEFITS SEEN OF MAGNET THERAPY ARE:

- *It helps alleviate pain and improve mobility of arthritic joints.*

- *Recovery of nerve sensation.*

- *It aids recovery of torn ligaments, muscles and tendons.*

- *It reduces bruising and swelling.*

- *It speeds recovery in sports injuries.*

- *Greater resistance to infection.*

- *It improves circulation/body and extremity warming.*

- *It helps removal of waste products from the blood, i.e. lactic acids, calcium, cholesterol and fat deposits.*

- *It increases energy and strength.*

- *It speeds healing, i.e. bone fractures.*

- *It helps recovery or can prevent onset of R.S.I./Carpal Tunnel Syndrome.*

- *It alleviates migraine and headaches.*

- *It improves overall health.*

If your general health is good, and you have no immediate areas to be healed, then by all means wear a magnetic bracelet. It is the simplest most effective way of compensating for the man–made EMF (electro-magnetic field) pollutants that deplete our systems. It will help to boost and support the body's own bio-energy system. Choose a 'north-pole' bracelet and make sure it is sufficiently strong to affect changes. My therapists and I all use bracelets.

HEALING WITH MAGNETS

Some interesting facts according to Dr Mark Atkinson BSc(Hons) FCMA FRIPHH. Although medical doctors and researchers remain sceptical as to the effectiveness of magnet therapy, recent research studies from major universities and medical colleges **have shown the benefits of static magnet fields in relieving pain.**

Below: magnet therapy aids recovery of torn ligaments, muscles and tendons.

The Office of Alternative Medicine of the Institute of Health, in Washington, D.C. awarded a million-dollar grant in 1997 for the study of what has been, until now, largely an Eastern and European phenomenon. Medical use of magnets is reimbursable by private healthcare in 50 countries worldwide.

Baylor College of Medicine, USA. Dr Carlos Valbona in 1997 published a double blind study of 50 patients who suffered from muscular or arthritic pain. Seventy-six per cent of patients treated with static magnets reported significant improvement.

New York Medical College, N.Y. Dr Michael Weintraub, a clinical professor of neurology, released a study in 1999 that showed he had significantly reduced foot pain in diabetics, by the use of magnetic innersoles in 9 out of 10 patients.

Vanderbilt University Medical Centre, found that between 80–90 per cent of patients with pain related to sports injuries and accidents found relief after magnet treatment.

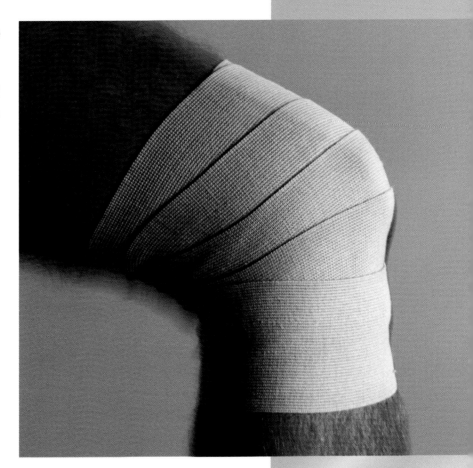

The Kouseikai Suzuki Hospital in Japan, in double blind clinical studies, showed that 83 per cent of their patients with sleep-related disorders benefited from the use of magnetic mattress pads.

One in three households in Japan are reported to sleep on a magnetic mattress pad.

BUYER BEWARE
Before you buy your magnets – the dos and don'ts of selecting the right kind.

Nothing is worse than throwing your money away on magnets that are no more effective than the ones on your refrigerator. It is what a lot of people are doing and, what is worse, they then say that magnets do not work.

MAGNETS DO WORK!

You just have to buy the best, and the best may not be the most expensive. Certainly I have seen some magnets on sale by multi-level marketers that are twice the price and half as strong as other reliable brands.

You must remember one or two key points in determining the right product to buy.

You have to remember the term **GAUSS RATING**.

The gauss of a magnet determines it strength. There is a gauss at the centre (core) of the magnet and one at its surface.

1. NEODYMIUM – THE 'KING' OF MAGNETS.
These magnets are made up of three metals: boron, ferrite and neodymium. Neodymium is a rare earth metal and expensive. The quantity in the manufacture will be directly reflected in the power of output the magnet will have.

Top-quality neodymiums will have a CORE rating of 12,300 and a SURFACE gauss of 1,200.

This magnet will have an impact of 3–4 inches on the skin both in radius and in depth of penetration.

They are called 'permanent' magnets and they will hold their fields for up to 15 years

These magnets should be used for most soft-tissue damage as they are the most likely to get the best results in areas such as backs, knees hips, shoulders etc..

I have seen some magnets on sale with a core gauss of 400. The surface rating is barely anything and it would be lucky to penetrate $\frac{1}{8}$ inch deep. Some of these are 'exhausted' after a few days and the manufacturer suggests you throw them away.

Make sure you understand what you are getting when choosing a magnet. Do NOT go for attractive packaging or ads. **Read the information, ask a therapist or call the help line.**

If the packaging does not tell you the strength (GAUSS, surface and core), DO NOT BUY.

Your results depend on it. The search for a good product does really pay off in the end.

2. A less expensive magnet is a **FLEXIBLE** one. A flexible is approximately 2,750 gauss at its core. This will have an impact on tissue of between 1–2 inches.

Flexible magnets are used for fingers, thumbs and wrist wraps, where less penetration is required. They are also available for backs and knees, but for these deeper areas I would strongly advise the use of neodymiums.

A flexible magnet generally holds its field for 5–6 years.

3. **CERAMIC** magnets. Ceramic magnets are generally found in pillow pads and sleep systems. Their gauss is 3,950 and they promote relaxation whilst you sleep. They also kick in the pineal gland (remember Cleopatra!).

Ceramic magnets are far less costly than neodymiums, and so manufactures can readily build them into large items, such as mattress pads, at a fraction of the cost that neos would be.

You will find most of the above magnets will have the NORTH POLE of the magnet towards the body. It is the general consensus that North Pole – Heals South Pole – Stimulates. For healing, most companies use north pole towards the body. Occasionally my therapists will treat a patient in their clinics with a limited exposure to south pole, <u>but the general rule I would recommend for you is to use north pole magnets only.</u>

Of course, there is always an exception.

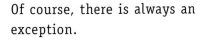

Innersoles:
Magnetic innersoles are usually used by patients and athletes who are looking to improve circulation, energy and strength. They are also used for foot, ankle and lower-leg pain.

Left: 1 inch neodymium magnets.

Below: innersoles are usually used by patients and athletes who are looking to improve circulation, energy and strength

Below: ceramic magnets are generally found in pillow pads and sleep systems.

4. Innersoles are usually **BI—POLAR and FLEXIBLE**.

They will probably be sold in two or three sizes (small, medium and large) and the customer will simply cut them down to size with a good pair of scissors. Magnetic soles will not take up that much room in your shoes, and the results are certainly worth it.

WRISTBANDS AND BRACELETS:

There are many varieties of these particular magnetic devices now hitting the market, and they are certainly worth looking at. Some are very pretty, but hardly effective, while some are pretty ugly but powerful.

So this is the question you must ask yourself before you buy.

'What do I want the bracelet to do for me?'

If the answer to the above question is pain relief in the hand or wrist or for your general health, or to help keep your blood cleansed, then buy a wristband and keep it on. It is a simple and effective way of achieving these things.

I wear one continually, as do most of my therapists.

Once again, insist on knowing the gauss, surface and core, and get it in writing.

Be sure of your supplier. A magnet of **less than 800 GAUSS on the surface of your skin** will give hardly any benefit. The one I wear has six small neodymiums inset in a stainless-steel link bracelet. The surface strength of each neo is 1,200 gauss. It is attractive, strong and powerful. That is what you must look for.

Below: this bracelet has six small neodymiums inset in a stainless-steel link bracelet. The surface strength of each neo is 1,200 gauss. It is attractive, strong and powerful.

If your answer to the above question is that you want the bracelet for pain relief in your knee, forget it. As I said, with directly applied quality magnets I would expect to see pain relief within hours/days. Many bracelet companies will give you a 90-day money-back guarantee. I presume this is because they think it will take that amount of time for the blood to circulate, cleanse the system of toxins and have an effect in the injured area. As a practising therapist, I would never treat an injured area in this way.

HOW TO USE YOUR MAGNETS:

By now I should have drummed it into you to apply the magnet to the site of your pain.

Buy a quality product. If you have absorbed most of the above information, you will now know how to determine this. The rest is pretty easy. Most good manufacturers will have done the work for you. They understand when building their wraps, e.g. for the knee, that the penetration may have to reach 5–6 inches into tissue. So they will give the wrap sufficient strength to do so. Manufacturers will not overbuild a product, so you may be sure they are safe for you to use freely as and when you want to.

Above: therapist's magnets.

Always be sure you have a complete understanding of what is troubling you, either by a diagnosis from your doctor or your specialist.

Towards the end of this book you will find a section on treatment methods. This has been compiled by Valerie Dargonne as part of our ongoing training programme.

MAGNETS IN SPORT

Two years ago a British Tri-athlete sportsman came to me and asked if I could work with him to improve his performance and whether or not magnets could speed the recovery time of the injuries he periodically got from the various disciplines (running, swimming and cycling). His nutrition and training regimes were fine so we looked in the areas of strength, energy and stamina. We decided to use the following items on him.

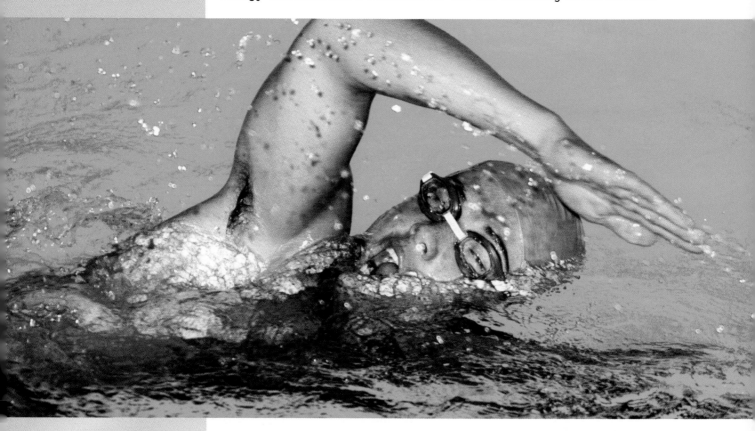

Above: magnets can help improve strength, energy and stamina, benefitting many athletes and sports people.

THE NEODYMIUM DISKS
These small disks are the size and weight of a 2p coin. Our tri-athlete could keep them with him in his first-aid kit and then place them anywhere on his body should he pull or strain a muscle. They would alleviate the pain and speed the healing process. We also suggested that he should use them on his lower back when he cycled to offset the normal ache he would get during the long cycling events.

A SLEEP SYSTEM
He took a single mattress pad around with him to place on his bed at night. The mattress pad allowed him to achieve a deeper 'alpha' state of sleep, to recover from the exhaustion of the day's events and wake with increased energy and without tired muscles.

SUPREME INNERSOLES:

The innersoles were used *after* his running races to *repair* the damage to the feet.

He also used the innersoles *during* the cycling events to add power and stamina to the legs. After a 112-mile training session he reported that at 92 miles he just left his team-mates behind. He knew that normally they were all pretty well matched. He re-tested them the following week and confirmed the extra performance the innersoles gave him. He now wears them for all his races.

I tease him that he is *cheating*. He tells me it's *ergogenics!* I regularly have both professional and general everyday riders using innersoles to great benefit.

There are now many top pro sports using them for repair in any sport which 'traumatises' the feet, prime examples of which are running and kick-boxing. The athlete uses the innersole in their shoes after they have performed to bring in the extra blood flow to start repairing the area and flush out the lactic acid that has built up.

For events that use a shoe that can take the extra sole and who do not require the agility of a runner such as skiing, skating, weight-lifting, golf and tennis, then the magnetic innersole is worn to enhance the performance. I have been told that **The British Federation of Ice Skating** is currently trying to ban innersoles as an 'unfair advantage'.

I mentioned earlier that many countries use them regularly. It is not new, or avant-garde any longer – just normal practice. We are only now becoming aware of their effectiveness in the UK. We now have calls daily from premier-league soccer clubs, golfer, rowers, weight-lifters and skaters to see if we will work with them.

The age of magnets in sport is here – ask the rest of the world!

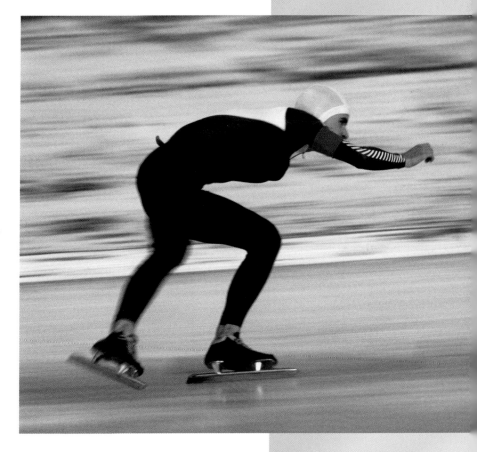

Below: the British Federation of Ice Skating is currently trying to ban innersoles as an 'unfair advantage'.

LET'S LOOK AT THE BEAUTY ASPECT

Below: magnet therapy can do wonders for the skin, hair and nails.

Almost a side-effect of magnet therapy are the things it can do for the skin, hair and nails. This happens because magnet therapy increases blood flow to the body. It is almost the same 'rush' as doing an aerobic work-out or, more specifically, having a massage.

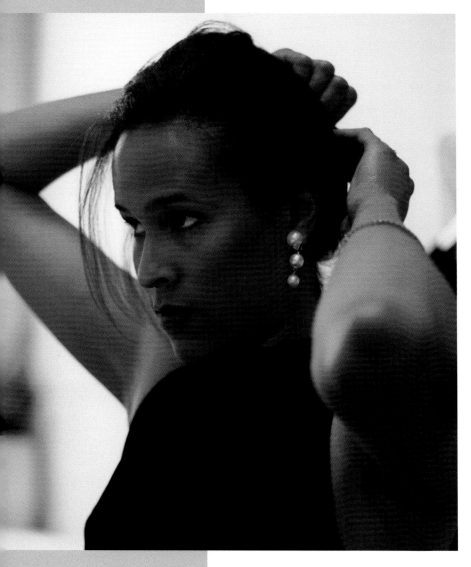

When you have a facial and the beauty therapist is massaging your face, 90 per cent of the work is the stimulation of cells and not the specific cream used. As they massage the skin the same reaction occurs as magnets produce, namely increased blood flow and lymphatic drainage. Now we all know how wonderful a good massage feels. There is nothing quite like it. Touch is so essential. However, consider having an eight-hour facial massage every night.

This is what happens when my patients use a magnetic pillow pad or sleep system. They may have bought it to ease stress or to promote sleep, but the side- effects are a radiant glowing skin, brighter and less puffy eyes and glossy hair. Of course you do not have to have insomnia or stress to benefit from a pillow or mattress pad. One of my patients, Fay, called me and complained that I was costing her too much money.

She had bought a lower back wrap for severe back pain, innersoles for increased energy, Neo disks and a pillow pad for stress. Fay then told me the products were not her problem. Her problem was that her hair was growing so quickly that she now had to get her roots tinted every four weeks instead of six! Sometimes you can't win.

Another client who had suffered badly from Carpal Tunnel Syndrome saw a great improvement in her nails and began to take care of them for the first time in years. She was overjoyed. A year later, when I met her again, she told me her nails were not so hot anymore. Because we had eliminated the need to wear the carpal wrap any more, she was not getting the extra oxygen to her hands. So she bought a magnetic bracelet from me, and has polished her nails ever since.

So a very simple beauty tip is to use a pillow pad. I buy one that fits an American king-size pillow which is 13 inches x 27 inches and I use it across my shoulders in bed and also on my car seat for long trips. A lot of my patients with arthritis use it in their chairs, especially for watching TV, or whilst at their computers.

NOTE:
It is quite safe to handle floppy disks, videos and your credit cards when wearing bracelets or magnets. Just do not put powerful Neos directly on top of them.

WATER, WATER, WATER!

'Is it that important?'

Yes, I promise you it is. Please drink a minimum of four glasses a day. The books say eight, ideally. If you can manage that, your body will love you for it. Personally, as one who considered a drink during the day as tea or coffee, I am happy to do 4–5 glasses. In the winter, try drinking it hot. I know it does not sound too good, but I promise you, you will get use to it. And don't worry – it is tea and coffee that are the diuretics. Take it from the greatest bathroom-seeker in the world, water helps to dilute the effects of caffeine. Now, my daily regime is to have my morning cup of tea, followed by a coffee and from then on, I am on water. I may possibly have another tea or coffee during the afternoon.

Just get into the routine – it's worth it. For many conditions we recommend drinking magnetised water.

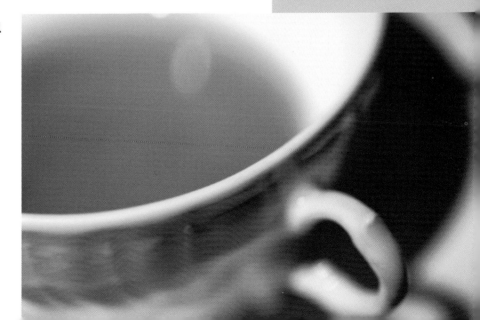

Below: water helps to dilute the effects of caffeine.

As a dancer I have grown up with the understanding that my body is my vehicle. It takes me from place to place, not my car. It is my body that gets me to the car or bus. Without maintaining this incredible machine, I am nowhere. It is the greatest piece of engineering I know of, nothing equals it and it is my aim to 'die, fit'. To do that I will feed it with good stuff (whole foods), exercise it and WATER it.

The rest is up to my magnets.

Since I have been using magnet therapy, which is coming up to five years, I have not had a cough or cold, my immune system is in terrific shape and I can also speak for my therapists and friends who use it regularly.

HOW TO MAGNETISE WATER

Any water can be magnetised. It is simple. Just place your jug or glass on a magnetic block for 20 minutes. It will then hold the magnetic properties.

NORTH POLE WATER: Place the container on the block with the North Pole facing upwards.

SOUTH POLE WATER: Place the container on the block with the South Pole facing upwards.

BIPOLAR WATER: Place a south-pole magnet on one side of the container and a north-pole on the other. Alternatively, mix the two above waters together.

Right: you can use Neos to magnetise your drinking water.

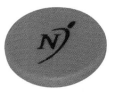

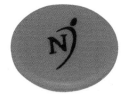

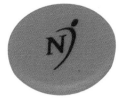

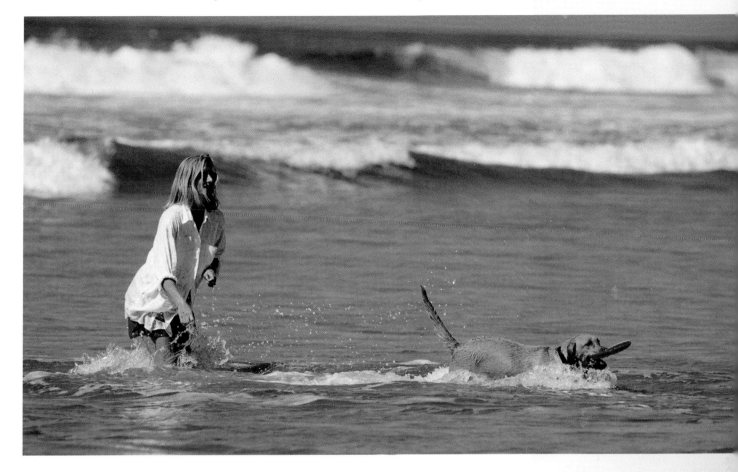

One of the nicest things we find with magnet therapy is watching the difference we can make to our four-legged friends. Getting positive results when dealing with animals is satisfying for two reasons. Of course, it is rewarding to help a cat, dog, rabbit or horse in pain – that goes without saying. The real buzz comes from the knowledge that the animal is not expecting anything to happen. When a dog with an arthritic hip responds because their owner has put magnets in their bed or on their collar, it reinforces our commitment every time. You will read about some of our work with animals in the personal testimonials

Above: magnet therapy can make a difference to our four- legged friends as well.

With animals, as with people, we can help with arthritis, oedema (swelling) and faster recovery from damage or operations. The horse-racing industry travels the world and for years it has been aware of the part magnet therapy can play.

You can find wraps for fetlocks, hooves and shins, and blankets, which help with the warm-up process before a race. The use of a magnetic wand is a great tool.

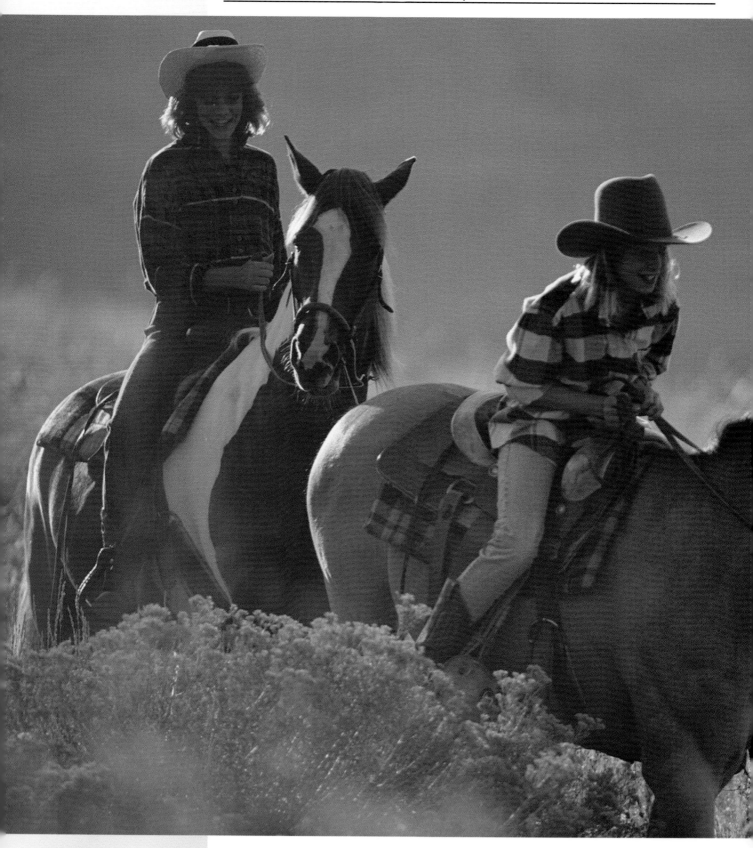

On several occasions I have worked with horses that were skittish and difficult to shoe. We found that by passing a magnetic wand (the Magnessage), which is a moving magnetic field, around the head for a minute or two, the horses would then calmly give their hoof to the blacksmith.

One little story I must tell you happened two years ago as I was driving back from a talk I was giving on magnet therapy. I was returning from Shepton Mallet to Bath when I noticed a group of people surrounding an animal at the side of the road. I could see the little creature was in spasm, so I grabbed my Magnessage and over I went. It turned out to be a small deer that had been hit by a car. The crowd had covered its head, not to shock it further and two men were holding its legs. Without touching the deer, I passed the Magnessage over it (the field of penetration on this is 15–18 inches) for a minute or so and the deer relaxed and stopped jerking. I then switched the Magnessage off and within 30 seconds the jerking resumed. Again I began treatment and she calmed down. I then carried on treating her until the RSPCA came. Unfortunately, her back was broken and she was put down. So even for a wild animal with its head covered something pretty significant happened as those waves penetrated her body. The onlookers were amazed and I had four customers before I got off my knees!

Time and time again my therapists and I see the healing power of magnet therapy, with the horses and domestic animals we treat. I have recently been asked to work with a tiger in a local zoo!

Once the word gets out about this treatment, magnets will be on offer everywhere.

Hopefully you will now be ahead of the game and know what to look out for and what to stay clear of.

Far left: with animals, as with people, magnetic therapy can help with arthritis

Below: it is rewarding to help a cat, dog, rabbit or horse in pain.

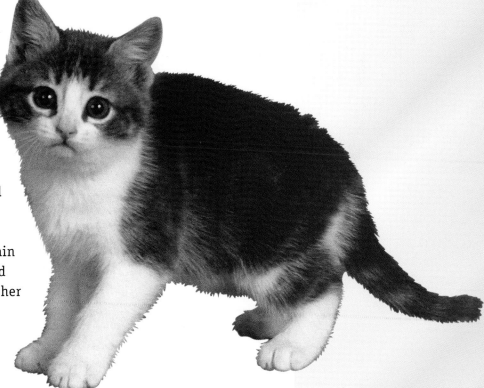

IN CONCLUSION – WHERE IS MAGNET THERAPY GOING?

It is my honest belief that magnet therapy will be available on the NHS within five years. Its part in relieving pain and reducing other symptoms in the areas I have described are too impressive to be ignored. By using magnets on people in industries where repetitive stress injuries are common, magnet therapy can offset the conditions arising, thereby saving millions in lost man hours.

Below: repetitive stress injuries cost millions in lost work hours.

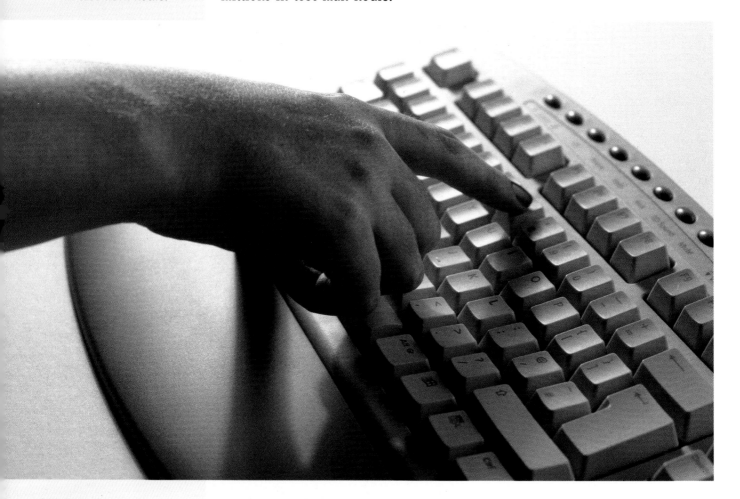

We are now entering a new era of taking 'energy medicine' seriously as the Chinese have for centuries. Even with the resistance put up by the drug companies and the Food and Drug Administration, Americans have over the last six years turned to it in their millions.
Yes, millions.

According to Jim Souder, the founder of Norso Biomagnetics, 'The modern magnets we use today are just the harbinger of where this technology will lead.'

From their clinics in the USA Drs Rosch and Lawrence have written, 'Although one would have to say magnet therapy is still in the formative stage, its future looks bright with promise – very bright indeed. One might even add that, as we are naturally attracted to healing and relief from pain, magnet therapy is pulling us irresistibly forward.'

So, as I mentioned earlier, know and understand the condition you want to treat. Feel free to share this book with your doctor or consultant. Most accredited therapists will be glad to answer any questions you may have. Further reading on this subject appears in the reference section of this book, together with some useful contact numbers.

For the sceptics out there I would say – you have nothing to loose, try it. All of us in magnet therapy would like to say: 'If it works, don't knock it.'

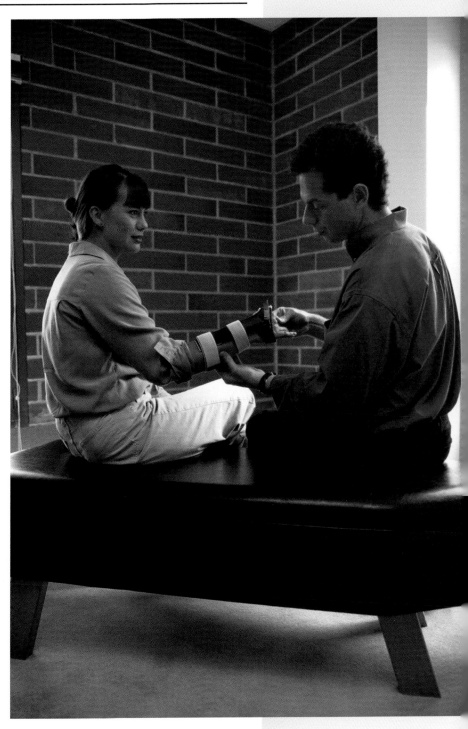

Above: 'if it works, don't knock it.'

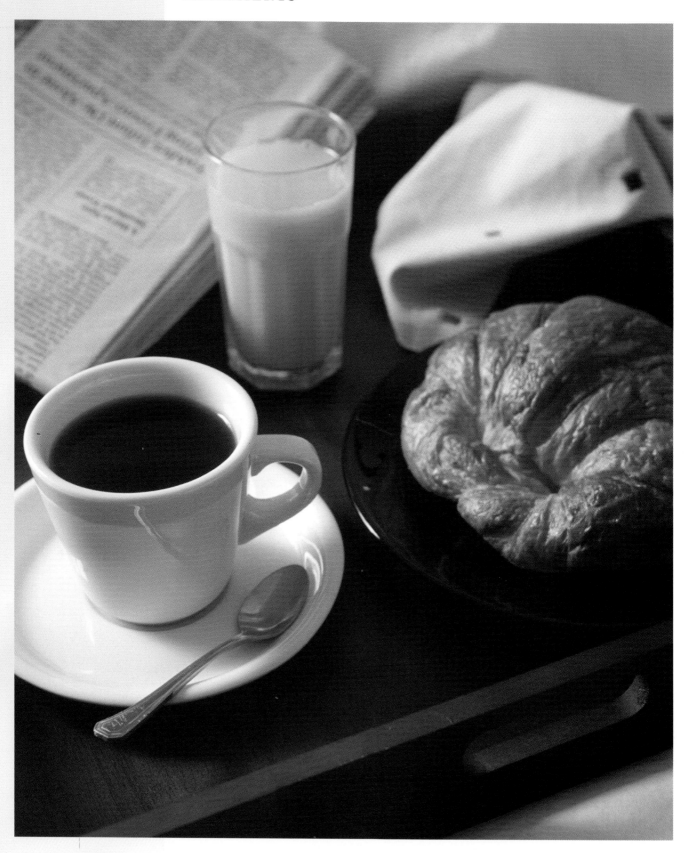

The treatments below have been prepared by Lilias Curtin M.C.M.A and are to be used as a guide only. For a more in-depth evaluation of a condition/problem, contact an accredited therapist as detailed in the back of this book or contact your local GP.

ACNE

Acne is a skin disorder caused by inflamed sebaceous glands producing formations of small pustules and blackheads.

Treatment

Sleep on a magnetic pillow pad.

Apply the north side of a magnet directly on the area for 20 minutes twice a day.

Drink north-pole magnetised water daily and use to wash skin.

ADRENAL GLANDS

The adrenal glands have two functions. One is the production of cortisone like hormones which help in the metabolism of fats, carbohydrates, proteins, sodium and potassium. Adrenaline is also secreted by the adrenal glands which prepares the body for 'fight or flight'. If these glands are not working properly, the patient will suffer from tiredness in the mornings, improving as the day goes on, hypoglycaemia (low blood sugar) and allergies, all of which worsen if large amounts of coffee are drunk.

Treatment

General treatment with a north-pole-orientated magnetic mattress cover, or magnetic insoles is recommended.

Apply a south-pole neodymium magnet over the adrenal glands for 10–15 minutes a day, followed by 30 minutes of north pole.

Drink south-pole magnetised water twice a day.

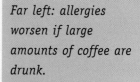

Far left: allergies worsen if large amounts of coffee are drunk.

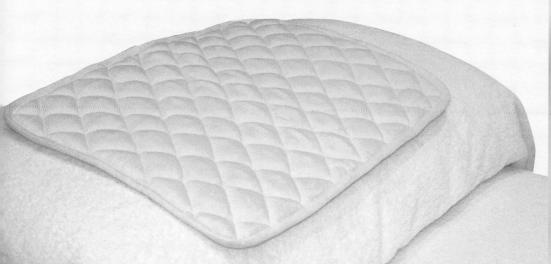

Left: a magnetic pillow pad.

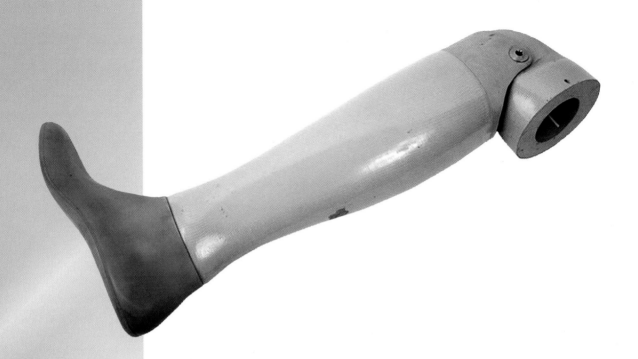

Above: some people with amputations suffer from phantom pain.

AGEING

Ageing happens to us all. The process by which the body replaces old cells with new cells slows down, leaving wrinkles and a weaker body. In very rare cases the ageing process begins early, sometimes even in childhood. This is known as progeria.

Treatment

General treatment with a north- - orientated magnetic pillow pad and or mattress cover are recommended.

Magnetic insoles may help to slow this process down.

Drink magnetic north-pole water daily.

AMPUTATION PAIN

Some people with amputations suffer from phantom pain where they feel pain in the area of the removed limb.

Treatment

General treatment.Use a north-pole-orientated magnetic mattress cover.

Sit on a magnetic pillow pad

Apply the north side of a magnet at the closest meridian point to the amputation.

Drink north-pole magnetised water daily.

ANKLE (BROKEN, SPRAINED)

A visit to the doctor or hospital is always recommended followed by rest, application of ice, compression and elevation of the leg when seated. The ankle may swell, become bruised and be very painful.

Treatment

Wear magnetic insoles.

Apply the north side of a magnet/s around the ankle until pain/swelling diminishes.

Bathe ankle and drink north-pole magnetised water.

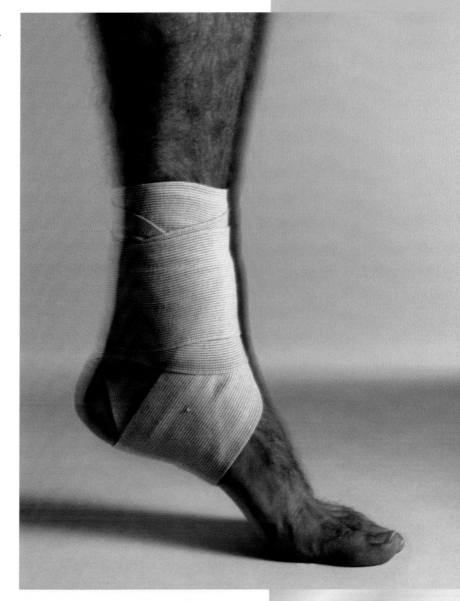

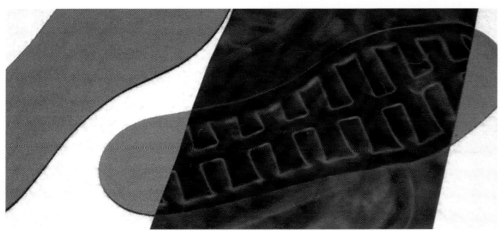

Above: a visit to the doctor or hospital is always recommended.

left: magnetics inside insoles - showing the placement of magnets.

ARTHRITIS

Damage or destruction to the cartilage of joints causes arthritis. The most common forms are rheumatoid arthritis or osteo–arthritis. The main symptoms are pain, swelling, stiffness, inflammation and formation of bone spurs.

Treatment

General treatment with a magnetic mattress cover, insoles or wristband can be used, depending on which joints are affected.

Apply the north side of a magnet or magnetic wrap to the area of pain or swollen joint.

South-pole magnetised oils can be massaged into painful joints

Drink north-pole magnetised water.

Below: for arthritis treatment with a magnetic mattress cover, insoles or wristband can be used, depending on which joints are affected.

ASTHMA AND ALLERGIES

Asthma is characterised by paroxysms of difficult breathing, giving a sense of suffocation. There is generally a difficulty in exhalation due to bronchospasm often caused by an allergic reaction. Other allergic reactions can cause hay fever, eczema and urticaria (hives).

Treatment

General treatment with a magnetic mattress pad is recommended.

Use the north side of a ½ inch neodymium magnet on a child's chest up to 12 years old or the north side of a 1 inch poker chip magnet on an adult's chest during times of difficulty.

Wear a magnetic wristband or insoles and drink north-pole magnetised water.

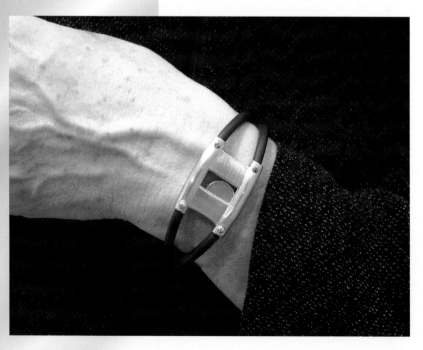

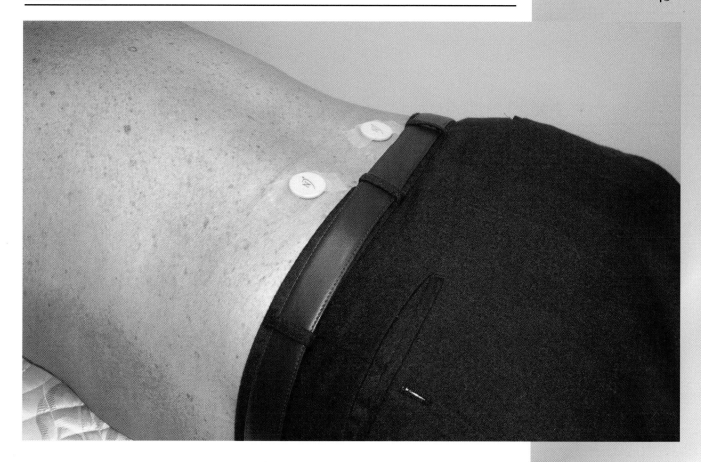

BACKACHE

Backache is not normally a serious illness, but can be quite debilitating. It can be caused by tensed muscles as a result of poor posture, depression or an awkward twist or fall. Occasionally it may be caused by gynaecological problems. If so, an examination by a doctor is necessary. Backache is one of the biggest causes of absenteeism from work.

Treatment

Strengthening and stretching exercises are recommended as well as correction of any bad posture.

General treatment with a magnetic bed can also help to alleviate the problem.

Apply the north side of a magnet or pad to the area of pain or attach a 1 inch neodymium magnet (north side) either side of the spine where the pain is felt. If the pain goes down the legs, apply the north side of a magnet to the back of the thighs at their highest point (under the buttocks). If the pain goes down the arms, apply the north side of a magnet to the shoulder joint.

Above: backache is one of the biggest causes of absenteeism from work.attach a 1 inch neodymium magnet (north side) either side of the spine where the pain is felt.

BITES AND STINGS

There are two major groups of stinging creatures: fish and marine life and some species of arthropods including insects and crustaceans. Bites can occur from all sorts of animals and pets including dogs, cats, horses, mice and rats.

Treatment

Medical attention must be sought first in case the bite or sting is poisonous.

Apply the north side of a magnet to the affected area until symptoms ease.

Bathe the area with north-pole magnetised water and drink north-pole magnetised water.

BLADDER PROBLEMS

Bladder problems can be split into two common causes – bladder infection (cystitis) or incontinence. Infections give several symptoms including a burning sensation on urination and increased frequency. Incontinence can be caused by injury to the nervous control or muscles of the bladder, leading to involuntary urination often during sleep or a coughing or laughing fit. Occasionally there may be an inability to urinate resulting in anuria or dysuria.

Treatment

Use a magnetic seat or pillow pad as a cushion.

Apply the north side of a magnet to both sides of the sacrum and also on the middle of each calf for half an hour twice a day.

Wear the north side of a magnetic pad over the bladder area on front or sacral area on back during the day.

Drink north-pole magnetised water.

Below: for bladder problems - Use a magnetic seat or pillow pad as a cushion.

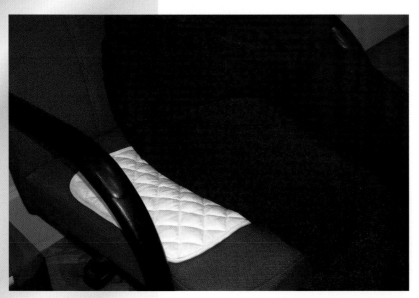

BLOOD PRESSURE

Blood pressure is the force or pressure exerted on the blood in millimetres of mercury on the upper arm, required to obliterate the pulse at the wrist. It is normally defined by the systolic (maximum pressure when heart pumping) over the diastolic (minimum pressure when hear is at rest). Average blood pressure of a healthy adult is about 120/80, high blood pressure is considered to be above 160/95 and low blood pressure below 110/70.

LOW BLOOD PRESSURE

Low blood pressure is not generally seen as a problem unless it falls so much as to cause fainting, Normally it may only result in poor circulation and weakness, in which case magnets can help.

Treatment

General treatment with a magnetic mattress pad.

Use a north-pole wrist band on the left wrist.

Drink north-pole magnetised water.

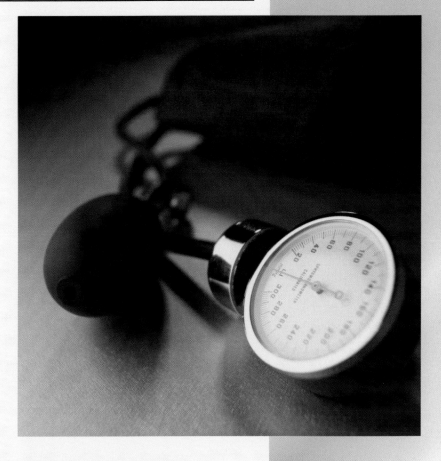

HIGH BLOOD PRESSURE

High blood pressure is, however, more serious as it increases the risk of strokes and other disorders.

Treatment

It is very important to see a doctor regularly so the blood pressure can be properly monitored.

General treatment with a magnetic mattress cover.

Use a north-pole wristband on the right wrist.

Drink north-pole magnetised water.

Above: high blood pressure increases the risk of strokes and other disorders.

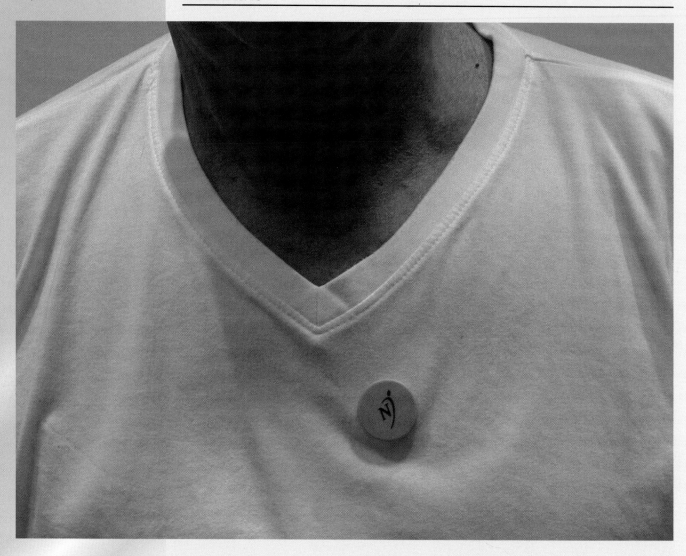

Above: for treating bronchitis apply the north side of a magnet to the bronchiole area.

BRONCHITIS
Bronchitis is the inflammation of the bronchial tubes by a virus or bacteria, resulting in a bad cough and fever amongst other symptoms.

Treatment

Apply the north side of a magnet to the bronchiole area during the day until symptoms subside. In bad cases a second north-facing magnet can also be worn on the back, mirroring the placement of the first magnet on the chest.

BONES – BROKEN OR FRACTURED

The skeleton gives shape, support and protection to the body. It is made up of 206 bones which are fairly strong but which can break or fracture if excessive force is put upon them. Once a fracture has been set by a doctor, magnet therapy can help in speeding up the healing process.

Treatment

Place the north side of a 1 inch neodymium magnet either side of the break until healed.

Bathe area with magnetised water and drink bipolar magnetised water.

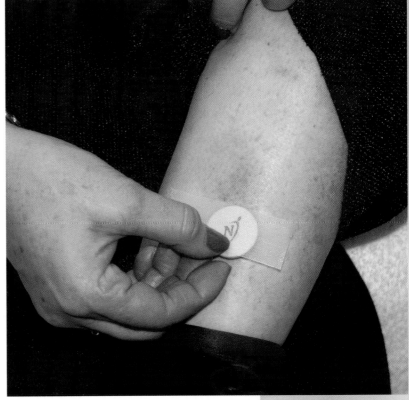

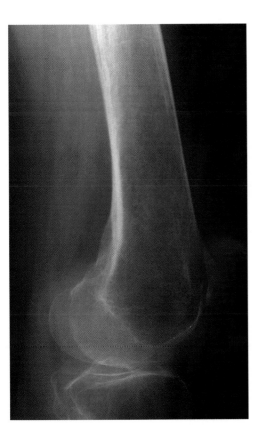

BRUISING

Bruising occurs when the skin is not broken, but the underlying tissues have been bleeding, leading to blue-purple discolouration. Bruising usually occurs after a knock or fall. It is not serious, but healing can be speeded up by magnet therapy.

Treatment

Apply the north side of a magnet or pad to the site of bruising or just above or below until signs of healing occur.

Bathe area with magnetised water and drink bipolar magnetised water.

Above: bruising usually occurs after a knock or fall; healing can be speeded up by magnet therapy.

Left: magnet therapy can speed up healing in broken bones and swollen joints.

BURNS AND SCALDS

Burns are classified into four different degrees, depending on the depth of tissue involved:

First-degree burns – the skin turns red;

Second-degree burns – the skin blisters;

Third-degree burns – the entire thickness of the skin is damaged;

Fourth-degree burns – show charring of the muscle and bone.

First- or second-degree burns must be held under cold water immediately, bad second-degree burns, third- and fourth-degree burns should be seen immediately by a doctor as these are life threatening.

Treatment

Apply the north side of a magnet to the site or just above or below if too painful until symptoms subside. Or use an electro-magnetic wand for five minutes three times a day to the area, replacing the magnets afterwards.

Drink bipolar magnetised water.

If any creams or ointments are used, magnetise them before use.

Below: for the treatment of painful burns use an electro-magnetic wand for five minutes three times a day to the area, replacing the magnets afterwards.

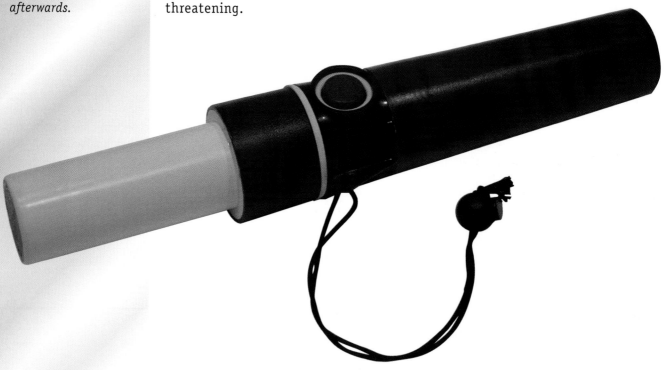

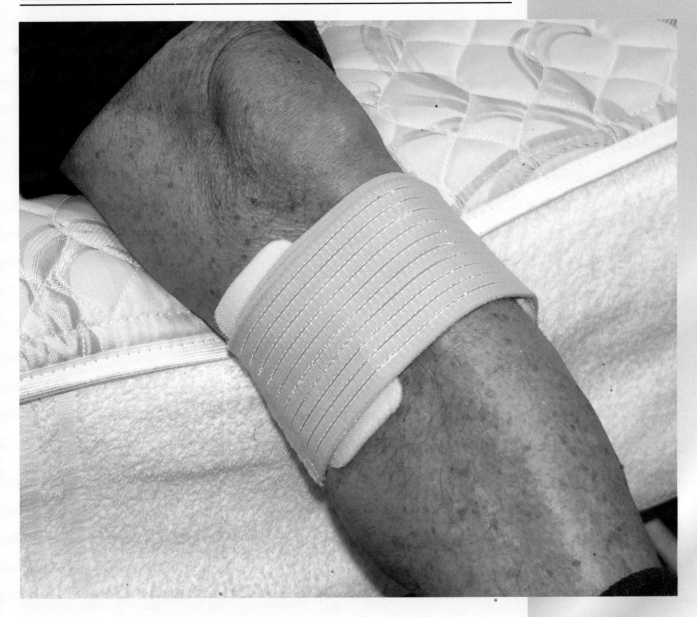

BURSITIS

Bursitis is inflammation of a bursa, a small sac of fibrous tissue filled with fluid between moving parts of the body.

Treatment

Apply the north side of a magnet or magnetic wrap to the area of pain

for several hours a day then increase or decrease periods as required.

Use a magnetic north-pole wristband.

Drink north-pole magnetised water.

Above: bursitis can be treated by applying the north side of a magnet or magnetic wrap to the area of pain.

CANCER

Cancer is one of our biggest killers. There are over 200 different types of cancer, and the one thing they all have in common is that a cluster of cells form a malignant tumour. Cancer cells have large and usually deformed nuclei with often two or three times the normal chromosomes. It is still not certain what makes the original healthy cell become deformed. There could be a variety of causes, such as radiation, alcohol, tobacco, asbestos and other such poisons. Viruses and genetic make–up are also suspected. In fact, there are so many possible causes and so many varieties that cancer has been a very difficult illness to prevent, diagnose and treat.

Treatment

As cancer is such a serious and complicated condition, magnet therapy should never be used as the only treatment or even considered to be a cure. If the cancer is caused by a virus, magnet therapy can help in improving the immune system thus preventing or even alleviating the problem in its early stages. It has also been recognised that cancer cells prefer an acidic environment in the body. Magnets neutralise acidity and render the body more alkaline, which makes it much more difficult for these cells to survive.

There is a lot of research going on at the moment with very encouraging results.

Russian research shows that magnet therapy, along with chemotherapy, has increased successes in treatments as well as causing fewer side-effects.

For these reasons we suggest a general treatment with a magnetic mattress pad with magnets which are north-sided to the body, and a bracelet to help the immune system and raise the alkaline levels in the body. Also magnets increase the amount of oxygen in the body. Cancer cells are known to dislike a highly oxygenated environment.

Drink north-pole magnetised water.

For specific problems call an accredited therapist or a recommended magnet product supplier's helpline.

CIRCULATORY PROBLEMS AND CRAMPS

The body needs a healthy circulation to keep warm as well as to function efficiently. Cramps can occur during exercise or rest when the muscles tighten due to lack of circulation.

Treatment

General treatment with a magnetic mattress pad is helpful.

Wear a magnetic north- pole wristband.

Drink magnetised water.
Wear magnetic insoles daily.

During a cramp attack, apply the north side of a magnet directly on to the affected muscle.

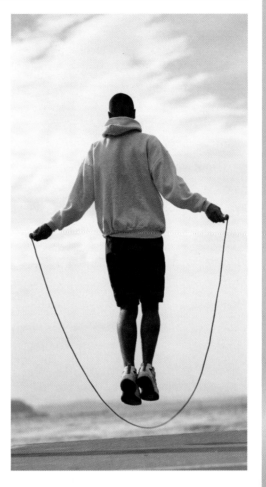

Left: cramps can occur during exercise.

Below: during a cramp attack, apply the north side of a magnet directly on to the affected muscle.

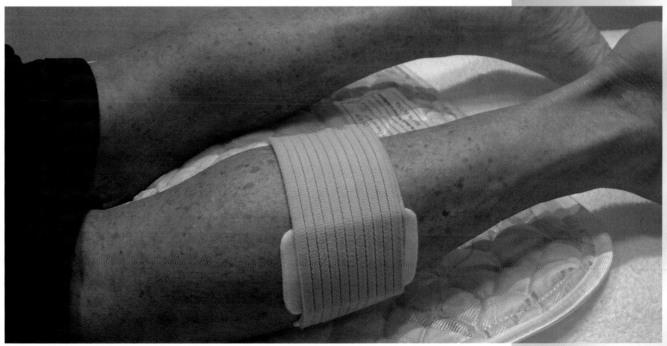

COLDS AND FLU

Colds and flu are unpleasant but not life-threatening. They are caused by a viral infection to the upper respiratory tract. They are caught when the immune level is low and not by getting cold as is commonly believed. There are several different symptoms including a stuffed-up or runny nose, cough, headaches and, with flu, a fever. These symptoms will eventually pass within a week. If not a doctor should be seen, as antibiotics may be required.

Treatment

General treatment with a magnetic mattress pad with magnets which are north-sided to the body will help boost up the immune levels, either preventing infection altogether or speeding up the recovery. Please note a magnetic bed must not be used for 24 hours a day. It is to be used at night time (8–10 hours normally). If you are in bed for longer periods, take the mattress pad off.

Use the north side of a wristband or innersoles to help boost the immune system.

Drink north-pole magnetised water four or five times a day.

COLITIS AND CONSTIPATION

Colitis is an inflammation of the colon due to an infection which causes chronic pain, constipation or diarrhoea.

Constipation is normally due to our diet and sedentary life styles these days.

Treatment

General treatment with a magnetic mattress pad with magnets which are north-sided to the body can be helpful.

Apply the north side of a magnet to the abdominal area as well as the liver and gall bladder for one hour twice a day.

Drink lots of north-pole magnetised water.

Right: for colitis and constipation treatment apply the north side of a magnet to the abdominal area as well as the liver and gall bladder for one hour twice a day.

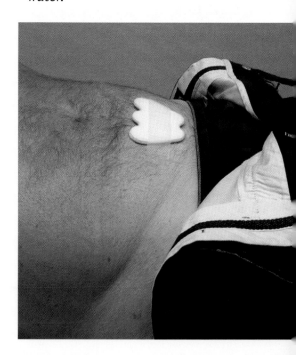

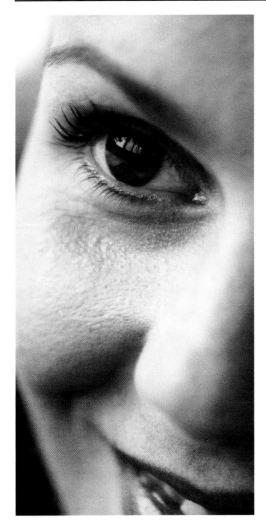

CYSTITIS

Cystitis is the infection of the urinary tract causing inflammation.

Treatment

Apply the north side of a magnet or magnetic pad to the kidneys, urethras and bladder during the day until symptoms subside.

Drink lots of north-pole magnetised water.

Left: treat conjunc-tivitis by washing the eye with cooled, boiled north-pole magnetised water four times a day.

Below: to treat cystitis - apply the north side of a magnet or magnetic pad to the kidneys,

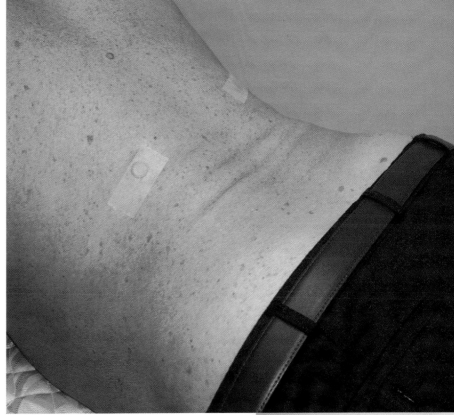

CONJUNCTIVITIS

Conjunctivitis is very common amongst children and is the inflammation of the mucous membrane covering the eye ball. It causes red eyes and a watery or yellow discharge.

Treatment

Wash the eye with cooled, boiled north-pole magnetised water four times a day.

Right: wear a north-pole wristband to help combat depression.

Right bottom: it is important to monitor the amount of insulin required during magnet therapy.

DEPRESSION

Depression is a common problem these days. It can be a result of several causes, the most common being stress.

Treatment

General treatment with a magnetic mattress cover with magnets which are north-sided to the body can help by promoting a deep, relaxing sleep and rebalancing hormones.

Wear a north-pole wristband.

DERMATITIS

Dermatitis is the inflammation of the skin caused by contact with external irritants, often dyes, metals, disinfectants and cleaning chemicals.

Treatment

Apply the north side of a magnet directly to the area.

Wear a north-pole wristband.

Drink north-pole magnetised water twice a day.

Wash area with north-pole magnetised water twice a day and apply oils or creams that have been magnetised.

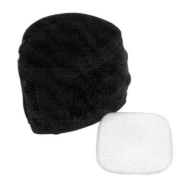

DIABETES

There are two types of diabetes – insipidus and mellitus. Insipidus is caused by insufficient secretion of antidiuretic hormone (ADH) by the pituitary gland and results in large amounts of pale urine containing no sugar.

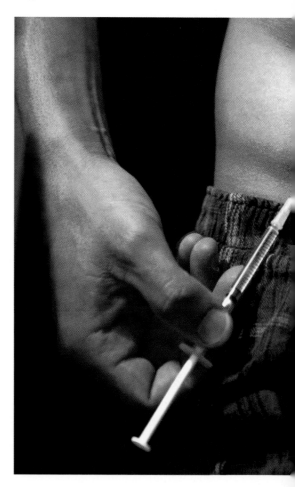

The more common form is diabetes mellitus, which is caused by the pancreas producing insufficient insulin necessary to metabolise carbohydrates. It results in excessive thirst and large amounts of urine containing sugar. If not controlled, diabetes can result in a coma.

Treatment

General treatment with a magnetic mattress cover with magnets which are north-sided to the body. North-pole-facing magnetic wristbands or insoles can help.

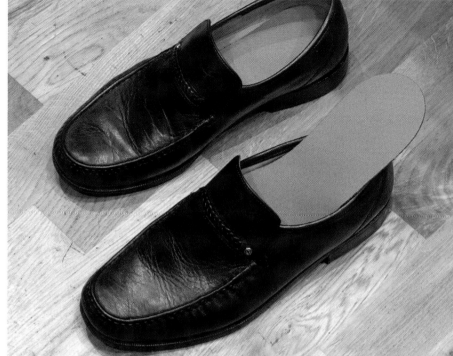

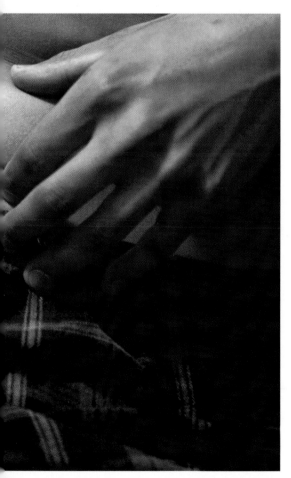

Apply the north side of a magnet to the pancreas and the thymus for 15–20 minutes twice a day.

Drink north-pole magnetised water three times a day.

IT IS IMPORTANT TO MONITOR THE AMOUNT OF INSULIN REQUIRED DURING MAGNET THERAPY AS THIS MIGHT NEED REDUCING.

DO NOT USE MAGNETS IF USING AN INSULIN PUMP.

Above: north-pole-facing magnetic insoles can help diabetes .

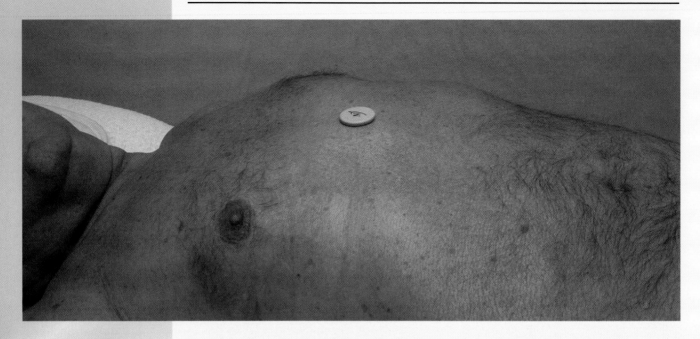

Above: for digestive problems (dyspepsia) apply the north side of a magnet or magnetic pad to the sternum area for 15–20 minutes twice a day.

DIGESTIVE PROBLEMS (DYSPEPSIA)
Digestive problems are caused by many factors, but mainly by poor eating habits and lack of exercise.

Treatment

General treatment with a magnetic mattress cover with magnets which are north-sided to the body is helpful.

Use a north-pole magnetic wristband.

Apply the north side of a magnet or magnetic pad to the stomach area for one hour before meals. It is important to remove all magnets from the stomach area during meal times and for a couple of hours during digestion.

Apply the north side of a magnet or magnetic pad to the sternum area for 15–20 minutes twice a day.

Drink north-pole magnetised water twice a day.

DIZZINESS
Dizziness can be caused by several conditions such as shock, stress, allergies but also by blockages in the sinus or ear canals. If the cause is unknown, medical advice must be sought.

Treatment

The north side of a magnetic pillow pad would be helpful.

Use a north-pole wristband.

Apply the north pole of a neodymium magnet behind the ear during the day.

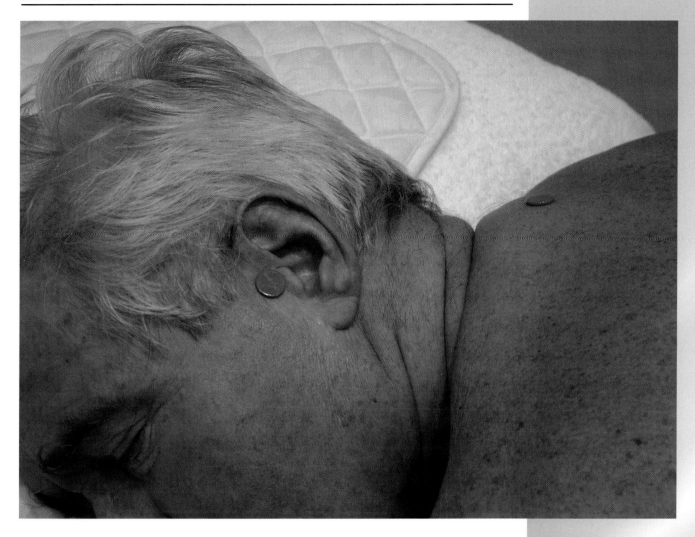

EAR ACHE

Earaches can be caused by several problems, the most common being a blockage in the ear canals.

Treatment

Apply the north side of a magnet or magnetic pad over the painful site, as well as over the seventh cervical vertebra at the base of the neck.

If symptoms do not ease, then seek medical advice.

Above: earaches can be caused by several problems, the most common being a blockage in the ear canals.

ECZEMA

Eczema is an inflammation of the skin that becomes itchy, red and blistered. It may weep or become crusty.

Treatment

General treatment with a magnetic mattress cover with magnets which are north-sided to the body can stop the night-time itches and accelerate the healing of the skin in general.

Use a magnetic wristband with north-pole magnets to the skin.

Drink north-pole magnetised water.

ENDOMETRIOSIS

Endometriosis is inflammation inside the pelvis and usually causes chronic pain at the time of ovulation and menstruation.

Treatment

General treatment with a magnetic mattress cover with magnets which are north-sided to the body can help.

Apply the north side of a magnet or magnetic pad to the lower abdomen for 12 hours at a time during these periods.

Drink magnetised water.

Below: for the treatment of eczema use a magnetic wristband with a magnetic mattress cover

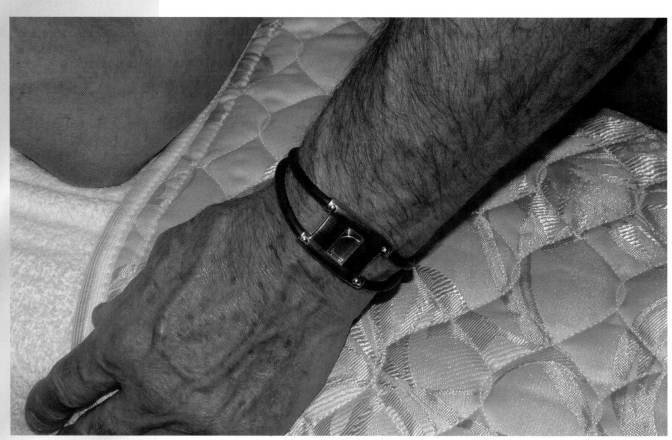

FATIGUE

General fatigue can be caused by a variety of problems – stress, overwork, lack of exercise, or lack of sleep.

Treatment

General treatment with a magnetic mattress cover with magnets which are north-sided to the body can help in giving deep-healing/energy-restoring sleep.

Wearing magnetic insoles or north-facing wristbands can help with fatigue during the day.

Apply the north side of a magnet on the thymus gland for 2–3 hours a day.

Drink magnetised water twice a day.

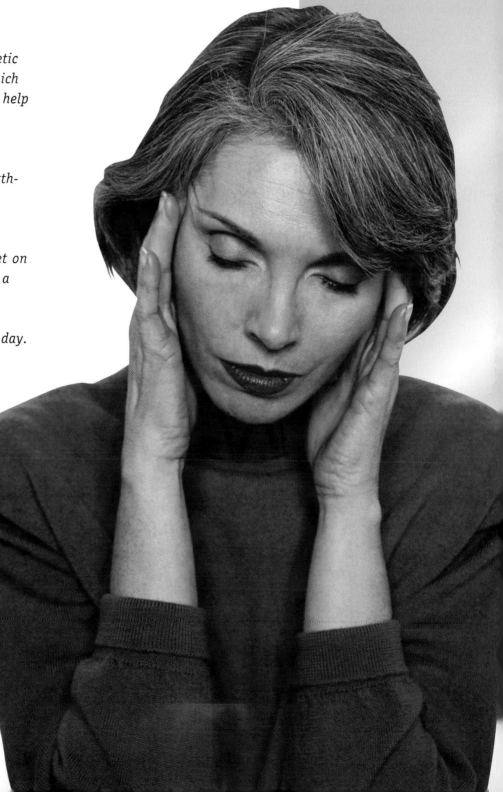

Below: fatigue can be caused by stress, overwork, lack of exercise or lack of sleep.

Right: fibromyalgia is inflammation of neck and shoulder muscles

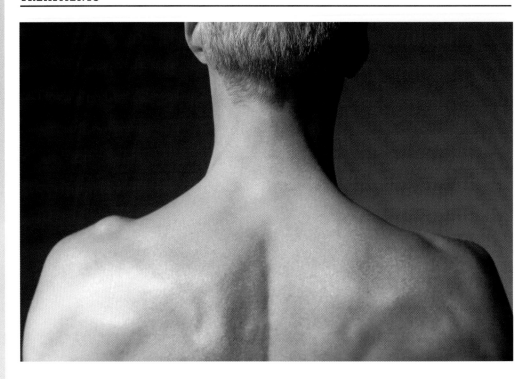

FIBROMYALGIA

Fibromyalgia is inflammation of nerves and fibres in the body causing severe pain in up to eighteen areas.

Treatment

General treatment with a magnetic mattress cover with magnets which are north-sided to the body and pillow will help in easing the pain at night, removing the acidity from the body and generally boosting the immune system

The use of a magnetic mattress pad will help to ease morning 'flare ups'.

Apply the north side of a 1 inch neodymium magnet over the painful areas.

Use the north side of a magnet on the thoracic area of the spine for 30 minutes twice a day.

FLATULENCE

Flatulence is gas in the alimentary canal, usually the stomach, giving bloating and pain.

Poor eating habits leading to the build-up of gas normally cause flatulence.

Treatment

Apply the north side of a magnet or magnetic pad to the colon for 1 hour twice a day.

Drink magnetised water twice a day.

FIBROIDS

Fibroids are tumours made of fibrous and muscular tissue which develop in the muscular wall of the womb.

Treatment

Apply the north side of a magnet or magnetic pad to the abdomen for 12 hours at a time for two weeks at a time when the pain is worst.

Drink north-pole magnetised water.

GALLBLADDER PROBLEMS

Gallbladder problems can be caused by anger or excitement combined with a poor diet, giving stomach cramps, nausea and even gallstones.

Treatment

In addition to a low-fat diet, magnet therapy can help in increasing the alkalinity of the body as well as aiding in digestion.

A general treatment with a magnetic mattress cover with magnets which are north-sided to the body is recommended.

Apply the north side of a magnet or magnetic pad over the gall bladder for 30 minutes twice a day.

Wear a magnetic wristband.

Drink north-pole magnetised water.

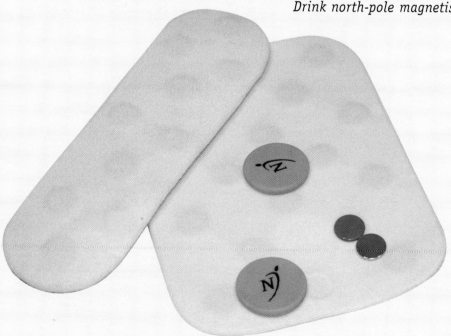

Left: therapist's magnetic pads, 1 inch and ½ inch neodymium magnets.

GLAUCOMA

Glaucoma is a disease of the eyes with a hardening of the globe due to an increase in the pressure in the eye. It can lead to blindness. The normal pressure in the eye is about 15. This can increase to 70 in a case of glaucoma.

Treatment

General treatment with the north side of a magnetic pillow is recommended.

Apply the north side of a neodymium magnet or magnetic eye mask to the side and below the eyes for 15 minutes twice a day.

Drink magnetised water.

Below: to treat glaucoma apply the north side of a ?' neodymium magnet or magnetic eye mask.

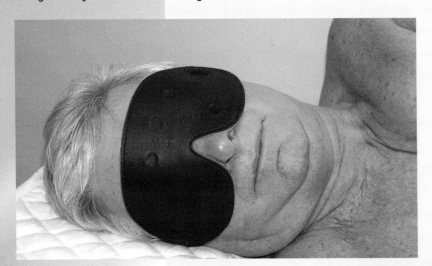

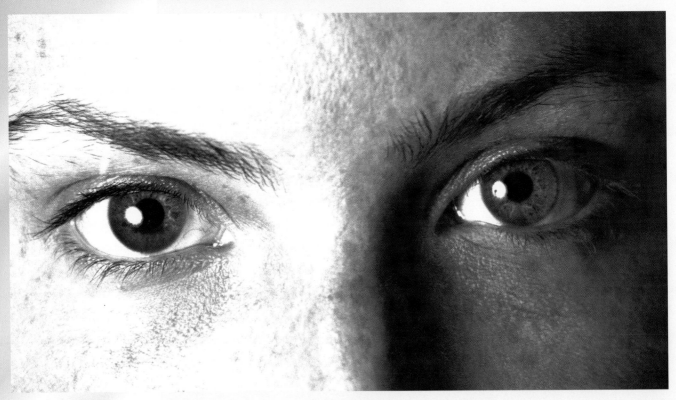

GOUT

Gout is an inherited defect of the metabolic system in which uric acid builds up in the tissues, giving swollen joints. Gout is often found in the toe joint.

Treatment

A balanced diet and gentle exercise are recommended, as well as magnet therapy to help reduce the acidity in the body.

Sleeping on a magnetic mattress cover with magnets which are north-sided to the body is highly recommended to remove the acidity from the body.

Apply the north side of a magnet or magnetic wrap to the affected joint.

Wear magnetic insoles if in the feet.

Drink lots of north-pole magnetised water.

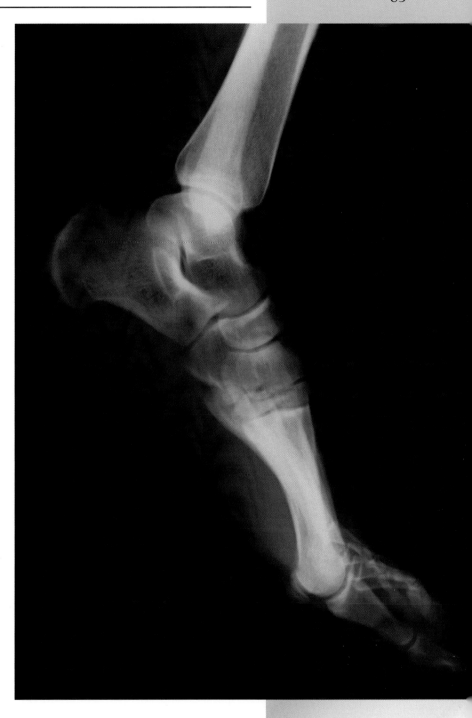

Above: gout is often found in the joints of the toes.

Far right: headaches are usually no more than a temporary discomfort.

Right: apply the north side of a magnet at the indentation at the outside edge of the eyebrows.

Below: relieving a headache using an electro-magnetic wand (Magnessage).

HAEMORRHOIDS

Haemorrhoids are veins in the back passage that fill with stagnant blood so the surrounding tissue becomes painful and swollen. Itching, bleeding and pain are normally felt during elimination.

Treatment

Sit on a magnet or magnetic seat for one hour twice a day. Gradually increase the duration to 4 hours.

Apply 2 x neodymium magnets (north-side), three inches apart, from the tip of the coccyx until symptoms subside.

Drink north-pole magnetised water.

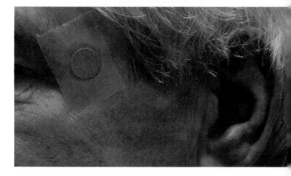

HEADACHE

Headaches are usually no more than a temporary discomfort, the most common causes of which are tension, alcohol, eye strain and changes in weather. If they persist, medical advice must be sought.

Treatment

Use an electro-magnetic wand (Magnessage).

Apply a neodymium magnet (north side) to the centre of the forehead and bitemporally for 30 minutes.

Apply the north side of a magnet at the indentation at the outside edge of the eyebrows, if eyestrain is suspected, for 15 minutes three times a day.

Apply a neodymium magnet (north side) on each side of the cervical vertebrae for 20–30 minutes three times a day if tension is suspected.

Drink magnetised water three times a day.

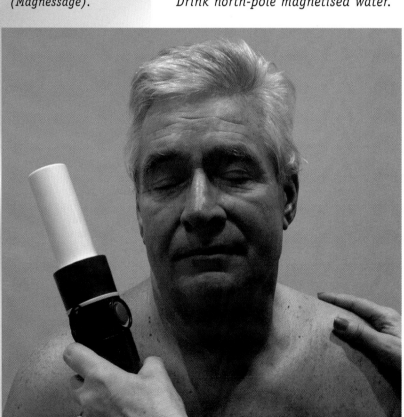

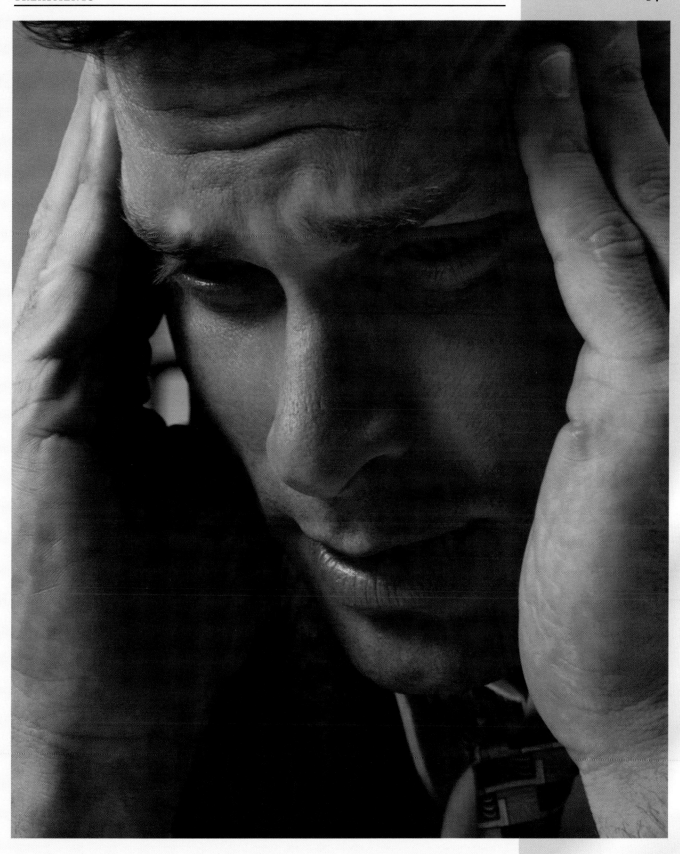

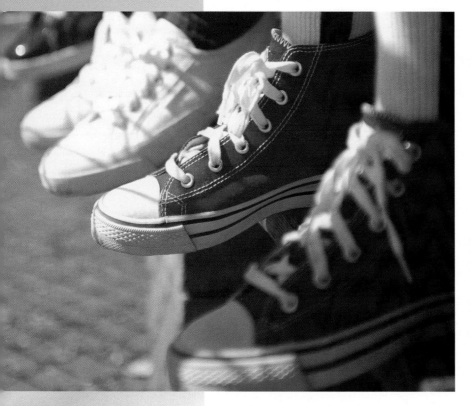

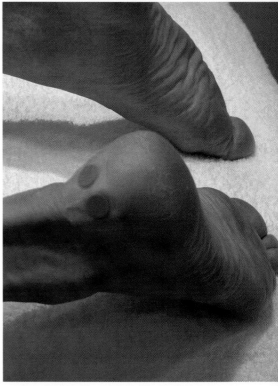

Above: heel spurs are a build-up of calcium on the bone of the heel, often caused by wearing ill-fitting shoes.

Above right: to treat heel spurs apply the north side of a neodymium magnet to the site and keep on for 24 hours a day for about two weeks.

HEART CONDITIONS

Heart attacks, heart palpitations and other heart diseases are generally caused by today's lifestyle of stress, tension, lack of exercise and poor nutrition.

Treatment

Wear a north-pole magnetic wristband.

Drink north-pole magnetised water.

NEVER USE THE SOUTH POLE OF A MAGNET OVER THE HEART.

NEVER USE MAGNETS IF A PERSON HAS A PACEMAKER OR DEFIBRILLATOR.

HEEL SPURS

Heel spurs are a build up of calcium on the bone of the heel often caused by wearing ill-fitting shoes.

Treatment

Apply the north side of a neodymium magnet to the site and keep on for 24 hours a day for about two weeks. If still painful after a two-day break, attach again for 24 hours a day for up to two weeks.

Wear magnetic insoles during the day.

Drink north-pole magnetised water.

HYPERTHYROIDISM/
HYPOTHYROIDISM

Hyperthyroidism is when the thyroid gland is overactive and becomes enlarged, forming a goitre. There are several causes, the main one being a diet short of iodine. Main symptoms are loss of weight and over-activity.

Hypothyroidism is when the thyroid gland is under-active leading to general tiredness, constipation and weight gain.

Treatment

Apply the north side of a magnet to the thyroid gland and another one to the base of the neck on the seventh cervical vertebra for 20 minutes twice a day.

Drink magnetised water twice a day.

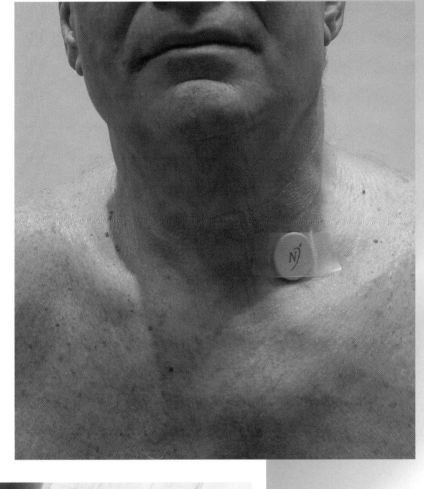

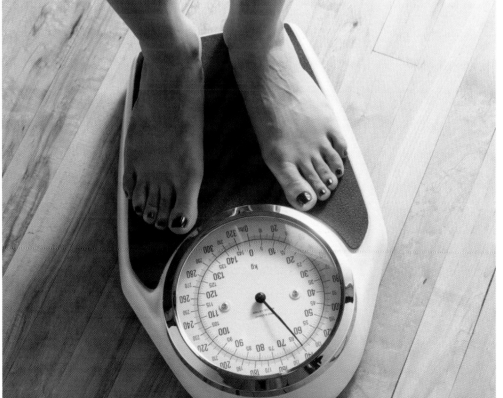

Above: for hyperthyroidism apply the north side of a magnet to the thyroid gland

Left: hypothyroidism is when the thyroid gland is under-active leading to general tiredness, constipation and weight gain.

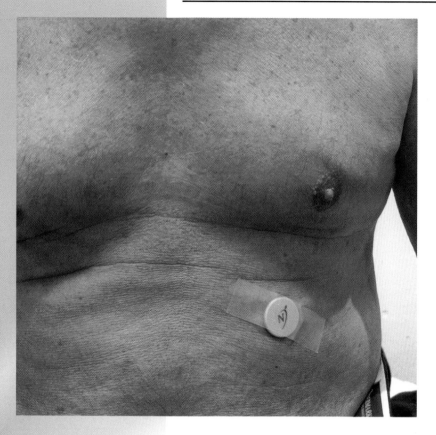

Above: to treat hypoglycaema apply the north side of a 1 inch neodymium magnet to the liver area during the day for a week and review symptoms.

HYPOGLYCAEMIA

Hypoglycaemia is a deficiency of sugar in the blood, which can cause cravings, mood swings and tiredness.

Treatment

Wear the north side of a magnetic wristband

Apply the north side of a 1 inch neodymium magnet to the liver area during the day for a week and review symptoms.

Drink lots of north-pole magnetised water three times a day before meals.

INSOMNIA

Insomnia is difficulty in falling asleep or frequent waking during the night. In most cases it is caused by stress, tension, discomfort or pain and can in time lead to more serious problems such as depression and exhaustion.

Treatment

General treatment with a magnetic mattress cover with magnets which are north-sided to the body and a pillow pad to help induce a deep alpha state of sleep as used in insomniac clinics in America.

Apply the north side of a neodymium magnet to the forehead and at the hairline behind each ear for 10 minutes before sleeping.

Drink magnetised water.

Also try to avoid stimulants such as coffee and alcohol for several hours before sleeping.

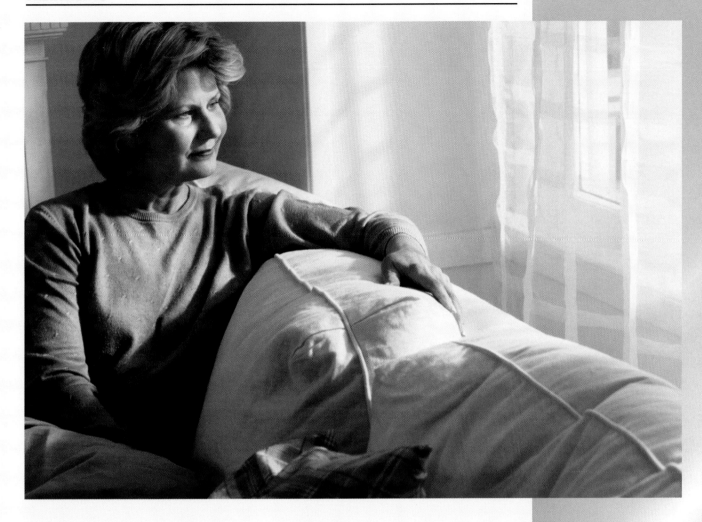

IRRITABLE BOWEL SYNDROME

Irritable bowel syndrome is not a serious problem, but can be annoying as it gives pain accompanied by constipation or diarrhoea. It is possibly caused by stress and tension or an allergy to certain foods. Try to eliminate foods such as dairy produce, wheat, yeast or sugars at different times from the diet to see if it is a food intolerance. Using magnet therapy can ease the pain and alleviate the constipation or diarrhoea.

Treatment

General treatment with a magnetic mattress cover with magnets which are north-sided to the body can help with food digestion and ease pain during the night.

Apply the north side of a magnet to the abdominal area three times a day (not during times of digestion).

Drink lots of north-pole magnetised water.

Above: irritable bowel syndrome is not a serious problem; using magnet therapy can ease the pain and alleviate the constipation or diarrhoea.

Below: menopause is when menstruation stops.General treatment with a magnetic mattress cover with magnets which are north-sided to the body will help to rebalance the hormones.

KIDNEY PROBLEMS

The kidneys are two bean-shaped organs about 4 inches long and found each side of the spine just above waist level. Their function is to filter the blood to produce urine, but because of our unhealthy lifestyle they have to work very hard and can malfunction.

Treatment

Apply the north side of a magnet to the kidney area during the day, until symptoms subside.

Drink lots of north-pole magnetised water.

MENOPAUSE

Menopause is the time in our lives when menstruation stops, usually at about 40–50 years. Hormonal imbalances often occur leading to mood swings and hot flushes.

Treatment

General treatment with a magnetic mattress cover with magnets which are north-sided to the body will help to rebalance the hormones.

Apply the north side of a magnet or a magnetic pad to the thymus gland and around the ovaries for about one hour twice a day, building up to eight hours a day when necessary.

Drink south-pole magnetised water.

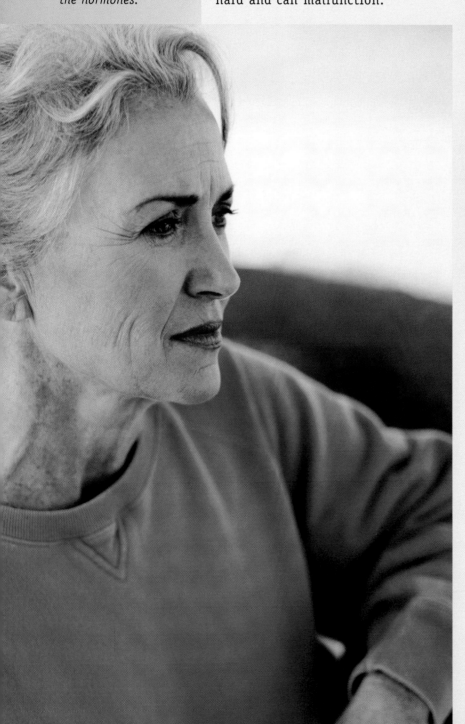

MIGRAINE

Migraine headaches are more than just a bad headache – they can be accompanied by vomiting and visual disturbances and can last anything from a couple of hours to a few days. The causes are varied – usually stress, tension or food allergies are to blame.

Treatment

Use an electro-magnetic wand (Magnessage) around the head for 10–20 minutes.

General treatment with a magnetic pillow pad at night-time or even during the day when relaxing.

Apply the north side of a neodymium magnet to the forehead or above the eye, depending on the main site of pain, for 20 minutes twice a day.

Drink lots of north-pole magnetised water.

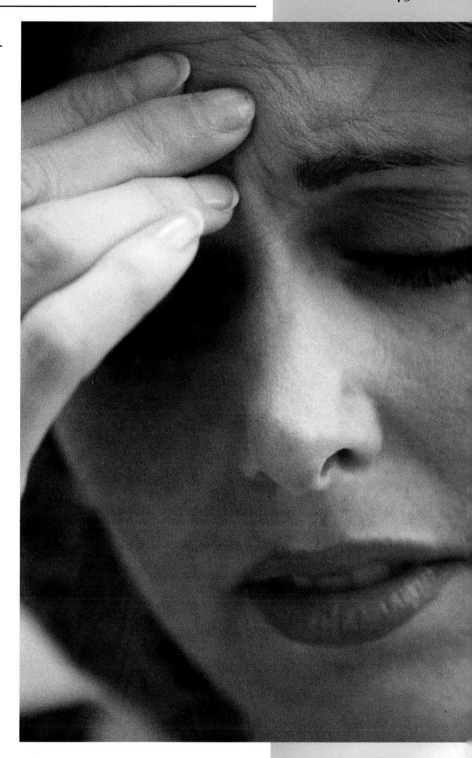

Above: Migraine headaches are more than just a bad headache.

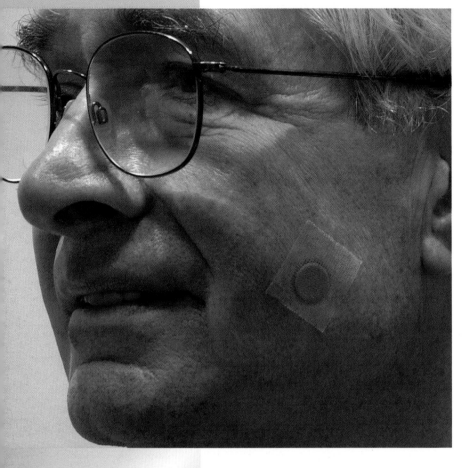

MOLES AND SKIN PIGMENTATION

The skin occasionally changes colour in patches often due to sun damage. Moles might even form which are raised areas darker than normal skin because of their pigmentation. They may also have hairs growing out of them. If they are very raised, become larger or bleed, they must be checked by a doctor for any signs of cancer cells. Once cancer is eliminated, they can be treated by magnet therapy to reduce them in size.

Treatment

Apply the north pole side of a ½ inch neodymium magnet over the area for about a week. If no improvement, leave if off for two days then re apply.

Above: the mouth can suffer from boils, abscesses, ulcers and cold sores. The treatment is the same for most problems

Right: for treating moles apply the north pole side of a ½ inch neodymium magnet over the area for about a week.

MOUTH AND TEETH PROBLEMS

The mouth can suffer from several problems including boils, abscesses, ulcers, cold sores and infections, all of which can be unpleasant.

Treatment

The treatment is the same for most problems. Apply the north-pole side of a neodymium magnet to the affected area until symptoms subside.

Gargle with north-pole magnetised water which has been previously boiled and cooled.

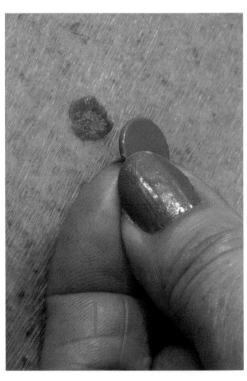

MULTIPLE SCLEROSIS (MS)

Multiple sclerosis, or MS as it is more commonly known, is a disease that attacks the central nervous system. The symptoms vary depending on which nerves are affected and how badly. It can appear at any age, but most commonly in the twenties and thirties. There are two main types, one which will continually worsen, and the other which can have several years' remission before another relapse. It is a very unpleasant disease with terrible symptoms and at the present time there is nothing much that can be done to help anyone who suffers with MS except to improve their quality of life.

Treatment

General treatment with a magnetic mattress cover with magnets which are north-sided to the body will help ease discomfort at night-time. This will also give more strength and energy to the body, whilst boosting the immune system.

Apply the north-pole side of a magnet or magnetic pad to any area suffering from pain, or treat symptoms as described under individual headings in this manual.

Drink magnetised water three times a day.

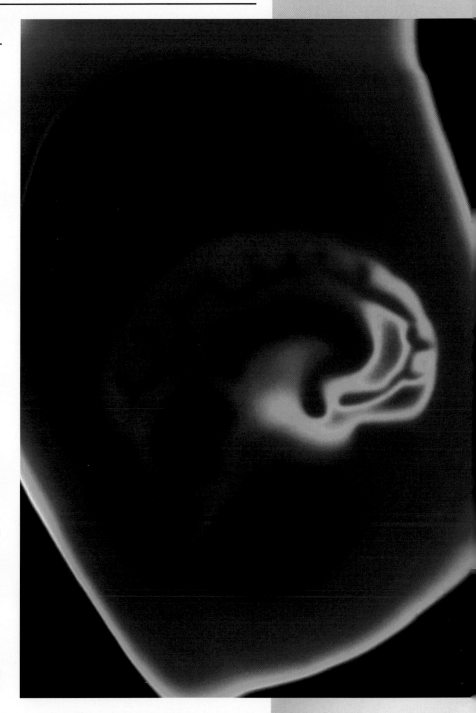

Remove or unplug as many electrical appliances from around the bed area as is possible. Do not use electric blankets.

Above: multiple sclerosis is a disease that attacks the central nervous system.

MUSCLE PAIN, SPASMS AND INJURIES

Muscles are specialised tissue which are attached to bones by tendon, which contract, resulting in movement of the joints. If these muscles are not used enough, they become weak and will normally only strengthen up with exercise. Magnets can help. Muscles can also suffer aches and pains due to over-exertion or a direct blow, causing build-up of lactic acid.

Treatment

General treatment with a magnetic mattress cover with magnets which are north-sided to the body will speed up recovery after excessive exertion as it removes the acidity from the area, accelerating the healing.

Apply several magnets using the north-pole side on the site to ease pain, or a magnetic mattress cover with magnets which are north-sided to the body.

Apply a magnetic pad over the sacrum area as this hits the meridian that controls the energy flow to the muscles.

Drink north-pole magnetised water three times a day or after exercise.

Below: for muscle pain spasms and injuries apply a magnetic pad over the sacrum area as this hits the meridian that controls the energy flow to the muscles.

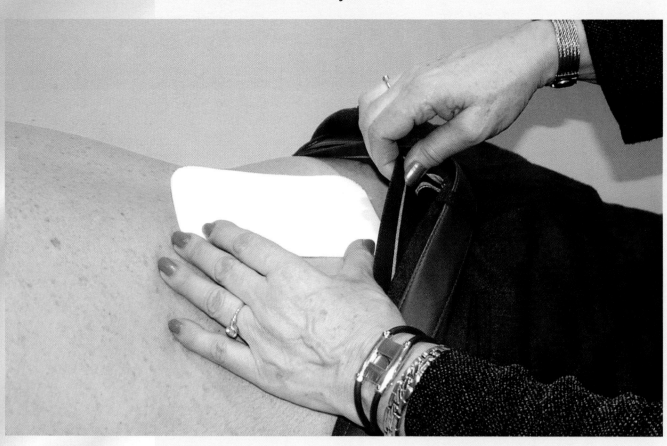

MYALGIC ENCEPHALITIS (ME)

ME, also referred to as 'yuppie flu' or 'chronic fatigue syndrome', is when the body becomes very weak often after an infection or virus. The person is more likely to catch any infection or virus they may come into contact with.

Treatment

General treatment with a magnetic mattress cover with magnets which are north-sided to the body will help with recovery and boost the immune system.

Wear magnetic insoles or a north-pole-facing bracelet during the day to help detoxify the body and give energy.

Apply the north-pole side of a magnet or a magnetic pad to the thymus gland for several hours twice a day.

Drink magnetised water twice a day.

Remove or unplug as many electrical appliances from around the bed area as is possible. Do not use electric blankets.

NECK PROBLEMS

The neck is an area affected by tension, poor posture and whiplash caused, by for example, a car accident. Tension from here can also lead to headaches.

Treatment

General treatment with a magnetic pillow pad can help.

Use a north-pole facing magnetic neck wrap.

Below: neck problems can be caused by tension, poor posture and whiplash. Use a north-pole facing magnetic neck wrap to help ease the pain.

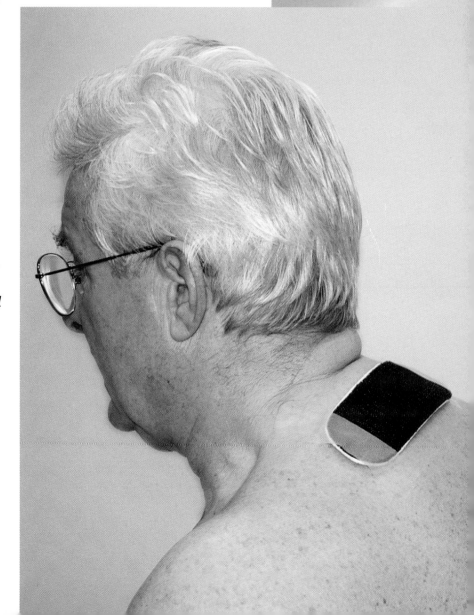

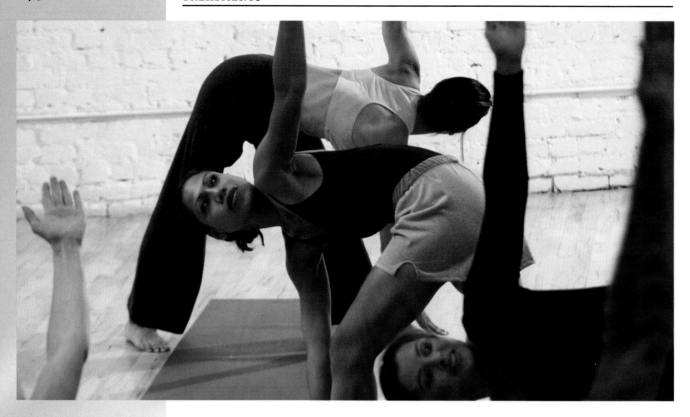

Above: a magnetic mattress cover with magnets which are north-sided to the body, insoles or a bracelet will help in speeding up the metabolic rate and giving more energy to exercise.

NEURITIS

Neuritis is inflammation of a nerve, resulting in loss of sensation and impairment of muscle control.

Treatment

General treatment with a magnetic mattress cover with magnets which are north-sided to the body is helpful.

Apply the north pole of a magnet or magnetic pad to the site of damage, or directly to the spine where the particular nerve is located for two hours twice a day.

Drink magnetised water three times a day.

OBESITY

Obesity can be caused by several factors – some fairly obvious such as over-eating and lack of exercise; others less obvious as they can be due to organs malfunctioning or even a disease or illness.

Treatment

General treatment with a magnetic mattress cover with magnets which are north-sided to the body, insoles or a bracelet will help in speeding up the metabolic rate and giving more energy to exercise.

Drink north-pole magnetised water to detoxify and flush out the system.

OSTEOPOROSIS

Osteoporosis tends to happen as we get older. It is the weakening of the bones owing to a decrease in calcium.

Treatment

General treatment with a magnetic mattress cover, with magnets which are north-sided to the body, insoles or a bracelet, depending where the affected area is.

Use the north side of a neodymium magnet or a wrap or pad directly over the site of pain as required.

Drink lots of magnetised water.

PANIC ATTACKS

Panic attacks happen for many reasons, giving a severe but short moment of anxiety, resulting in exhaustion.

Symptoms vary, but can include difficulty with breathing, sweating, dizziness, palpitations and nausea.

Treatment

General treatment with a magnetic mattress cover with magnets which are north-sided to the body, insoles or a wristband.

Drink lots of north-pole magnetised water.

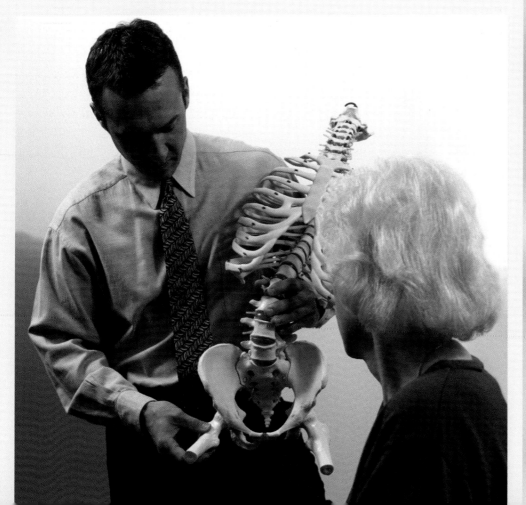

Left: osteoporosis is a weakness of the bones owing to a decrease in calcium.

PARALYSIS

Paralysis is the loss of power or sensation to the muscles owing to disease or injury.

Treatment

The treatment depends on which part of the body is affected.

General treatment with a magnetic mattress cover, with magnets which are north-sided to the body, insoles or a wristband, depending on the area affected.

Apply the north-pole side of a magnet, wrap or pad to the affected area.

Drink magnetised water twice a day.

PERIODS

DYSMENORRHOEA

Dysmenorrhoea is painful or difficult periods, often occurring during puberty or menopause. Medical advice should be sought first as there could be a serious underlying problem causing the pain. If, however, it is the normal discomfort felt for the first few hours or days of a period, a hot water bottle or a magnet therapy may be all that is required to ease the symptoms.

Treatment

General treatment with the north-pole side of a magnet, or pad placed on the lower abdomen or lower back can help in mild cases.

Apply the north-pole side of a magnet over the lower abdomen at night for a week before the period starts and until pain stops once started.

Drink north-pole magnetised water twice a day.

Below: drink magnetised water.

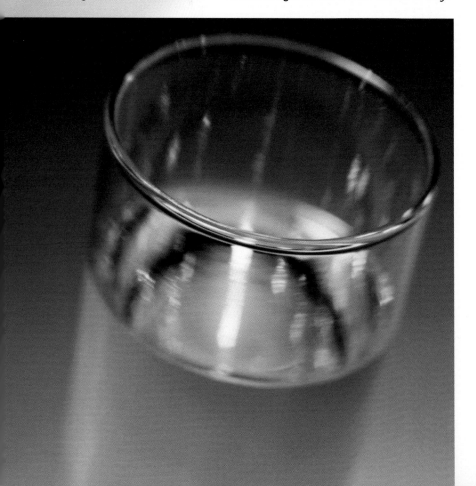

AMENORRHOEA

Amenorrhoea is the absence of periods where periods may never have started or when they stop for no known reason. It has a variety of causes, among them anaemia, stress and excessive loss of weight. There can be more serious causes and it is advisable to seek medical advice if the cause is not known before commencing any treatment.

Treatment

General treatment with a magnetic mattress cover with magnets which are north-sided to the body, insoles or a pad placed over the lower abdomen or lower back will help.

Apply the north pole of a magnet over the lower abdomen at night.

Apply the north pole of a magnet to the right foot and the south pole to the left foot for 20 minutes twice a day.

Drink south-pole magnetised water twice a day.

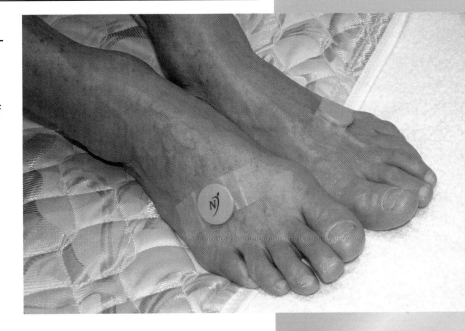

POST POLIO SYNDROME

Several years after a patient has suffered from polio they may experience muscle tenderness and pain, which is called post polio syndrome. Magnet therapy has had good results in alleviating these pains. The actor Anthony Hopkins used them on his pains and declared they were the answer to his prayers.

Treatment

General treatment with a magnetic mattress cover with magnets which are north-sided to the body, insoles or a wristband can help if a large area of the body is affected.

Apply the north-pole side of a magnet or magnetic pad to the site of the pain.

Drink bipolar magnetised water.

Above: to treat amenorrhoea apply the north pole of a magnet to the right foot and the south pole to the left foot for 20 minutes twice a day.

PRE MENSTRUAL SYNDROME (PMS)/TENSION (PMT)

Pre menstrual syndrome usually occurs a few days before a period is due. The symptoms vary from bloatedness and swelling to mood swings, fatigue and clumsiness. It is thought to be caused by hormonal imbalances.

Treatment

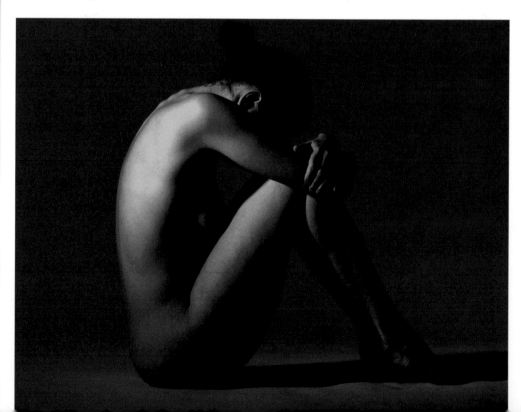

General treatment with a magnetic mattress cover with magnets which are north-sided to the body, insoles or awristband will help to balance the hormones.

Apply the north-pole side of a magnet to the base of the neck.

Drink bipolar magnetised water twice a day.

Right: pre menstrual syndrome usually occurs a few days before a period is due.

PSORIASIS

Psoriasis is raised itchy red patches on the skin mainly on the elbows knees and scalp but also on the hands and body. It is believed to be a result of a disturbance in skin enzymes.

Treatment

General treatment with a magnetic mattress cover with magnets which are north-sided to the body, insoles or a wristband, depending on the affected areas.

Drink north-pole magnetised water twice a day.

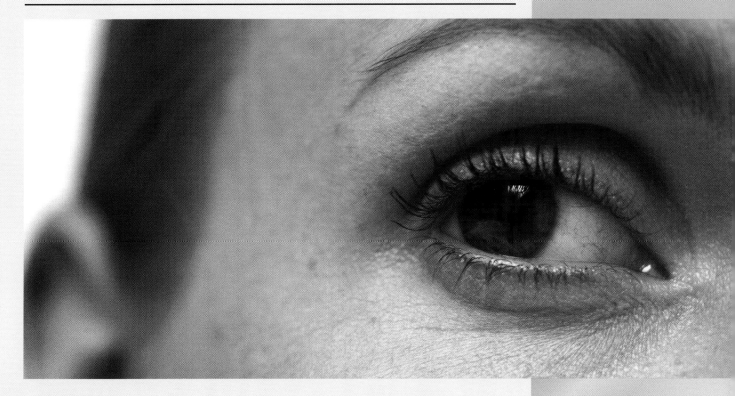

RHEUMATISM

Rheumatism is the general term for various diseases of the musculo-skeletal system. Characterised by pain and stiffness, it is often exacerbated by stress or cold conditions.

Treatment

General treatment with a magnetic mattress cover with magnets which are north-sided to the body can help if the problem is affecting several joints.

Apply the north-pole side of a magnet, or magnetic wrap to the area of the affected joint.

Drink north-pole magnetised water.

RETINITIS PIGMENTOSA

Retinitis pigmentosa is a degenerative disease of the eye, leading to eventual blindness. It starts with loss of peripheral sight, leading to tunnel vision and progressing to leave a small area of vision. It affects night vision as well as vision in very bright conditions, and it slows down the eye's adaptation to different light.

Treatment

General treatment with a magnetic mattress cover with magnets which are north-sided to the body, a pillow pad and insoles.

Wear a magnetic eye pad when resting.

Above: retinitis pigmentosa is a degenerative disease of the eye.

SCAR TISSUE

Scar tissue consists of fibres which are covered by an imperfect formation of cells.

Treatment

General treatment with a magnetic mattress cover with magnets which are north-sided to the body.

Apply the north side of a magnet or magnetic pad over the scar tissue during the day or night whichever is easier.

Drink north-pole magnetised water.

Bathe the scar in boiled, cooled magnetised water twice a day.

SCIATICA

Sciatica is a pain, numbness or burning sensation felt down one leg. The pain stems from the lower spine where the sciatic nerve is pinched by the two vertebrae either side of it.

Treatment

General treatment with a magnetic mattress cover with magnets which are north-sided to the body and insoles.

Apply the north side of a magnet up the leg where the pain is felt, behind the knee and just below the gluteal muscles as well as on the base of the spine.

Drink magnetised water.

Massage south-pole magnetised oil into painful area.

Below: sciatica is a pain, numbness or burning sensation down one leg. Apply the north side of a magnet up the leg where the pain is felt, behind the knee and just below the gluteal muscles as well as on the base of the spine.

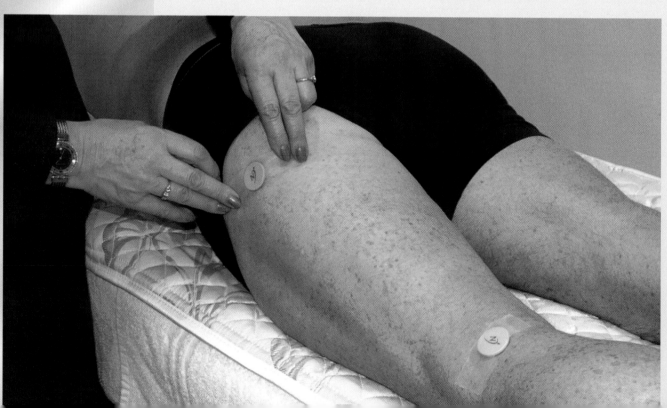

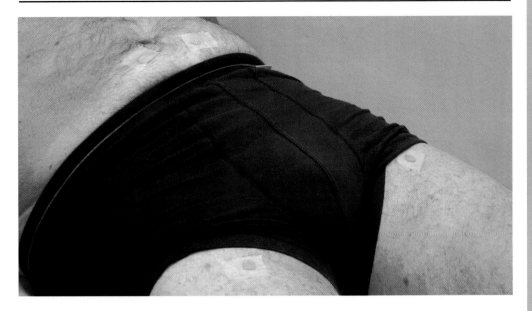

Left: for treating sexual problems apply two magnets (north-pole side) just below the navel, and two more midway down the inside of the thighs for 15–20 minutes twice a day.

SEXUAL PROBLEMS

Sexual problems are one of the most hidden and common worries. They can be caused by stress and tension.

Treatment

General treatment with a magnetic mattress cover with magnets which are north-sided to the body can help with relaxation.

Apply two magnets (north-pole side) just below the navel, and two more midway down the inside of the thighs for 15–20 minutes twice a day.

Drink magnetised water twice a day.

The use of an electro-magnetic wand (Magnessage) has proved to be beneficial.

SHINGLES

Shingles is a viral infection caused by the same virus responsible for chicken pox. The symptoms are a rash preceded by pain and skin irritation, usually along the course of a nerve.

Treatment

General treatment with a magnetic mattress cover with magnets which are north-sided to the body, a wristband and/or insoles will boost the immune system and remove the acidity from the body.

Apply the north-pole side of a magnet or pad to the affected area during the day.

Drink north-pole magnetised water twice a day.

Bathe area with north-pole magnetised water twice a day.

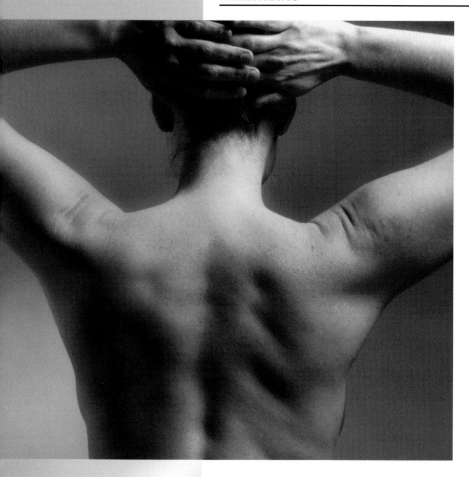

Above: shoulder pain often occurs due to stress and tension or bad posture.

Right: to teat sinusitis apply the north-pole side of a ½ inch neodymium magnet to the right side of the nose, and a south pole to the left side of the nose for 10 minutes twice a day.

SHOULDER PAIN

Shoulder pain often occurs due to stress and tension or bad posture.

Treatment

General treatment with a magnetic mattress cover with magnets which are north-sided to the body, and a pillow pad will ease the pain at night.

Apply a magnetic pad or 1 inch neodymium magnet (north-pole side) to the site.

Massage south-pole magnetised oil into the area.

SINUSITIS

The sinuses are cavities in the bones of the face and skull which reduce the weight of the skull and also add resonance to the voice. The sinuses that connect to the nose can become blocked and infected, causing pain and tenderness with a thick nasal discharge.

Treatment

Sleep on a magnetic pillow.

Apply the north pole of a 1 inch neodymium magnet to the forehead for 10 minutes twice a day

Apply the north-pole side of a ½ inch neodymium magnet to the right side of the nose, and a south pole to the left side of the nose for 10 minutes twice a day.

Drink north-pole magnetised water twice a day.

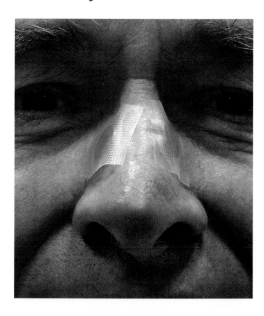

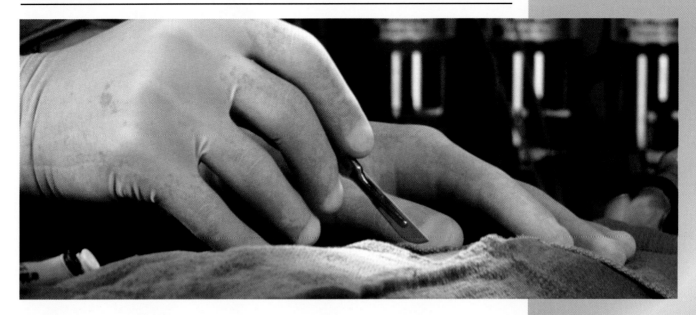

SPRAINS AND STRAINS

When ligaments are over-stretched some of the fibres can tear. This is called a sprain. When some muscle fibres tear, this is called a strain. Treatment for both is the same. The usual treatment of rest, ice and elevation of the affected area is recommended for the first 24 hours. Add to this magnet therapy and the treatment time can be halved.

Treatment

Apply the north-pole side of a magnet or magnetic pad to the area for a week during the day or until pain and swelling goes.

Massage south-pole magnetised oil into the area twice a day.

Use an electro-magnetic device (a Magnessage) on the area for five minutes twice a day.

SURGERY

Surgery has to be performed for many problems. Magnet therapy can help in accelerating the recovery time.

Treatment

Apply the north-pole side of neodymium magnets or a magnetic pad to the area for 48 hours before surgery.

Apply the north-pole side of neodymium magnets over the wound 48 hours after surgery to speed up healing.

DO NOT USE MAGNETS IN THIS WAY AFTER HEART SURGERY OR IMPLANTS. THE BODY WILL REQUIRE TIME TO GET USED TO THE FOREIGN MATERIALS. CALL A THERAPIST OR RELIABLE MAGNETIC SUPPLIER'S HOT LINE FOR ADVICE.

Above: surgery has to be performed for many problems.

Below: tennis elbow is inflammation at the tendon-muscle attachment on the outside of the elbow.

TENNIS ELBOW

Tennis elbow is inflammation at the tendon-muscle attachment on the outside of the elbow, usually caused by a repetitive, one-sided motion or over-exertion of the elbow.

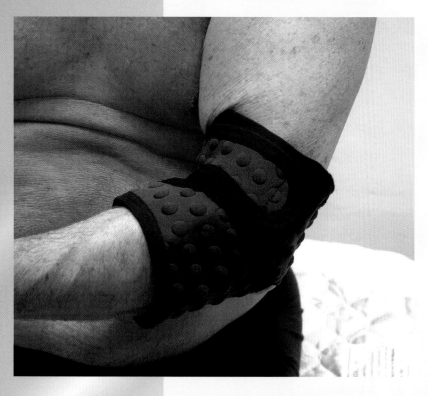

Treatment

Wear a magnetic elbow wrap, or attach the north- pole side of two neodymium magnets either side of the joint for 2–4 hours. Increase or lessen time as required.

Massage in south-pole magnetised oil.

Drink magnetised water twice a day.

TENSION AND STRESS

Unfortunately our lifestyles today are producing more and more tension and stress, leading to a multitude of other more serious conditions. If we can work on easing this tension, we might be able to alleviate several other problems.

Treatment

General treatment with a magnetic mattress cover with magnets which are north-sided to the body or a pillow pad are the most effective interventions. Magnetic insoles or a wristband will also help.

Apply several magnets (north-pole side) or a magnetic pad to the areas where most tension is felt, usually the shoulders or lower back.

Drink magnetised water twice a day.

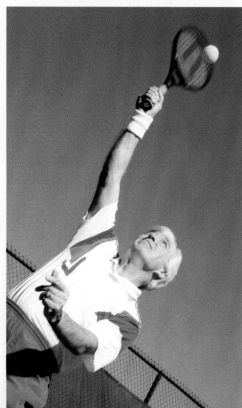

THROAT

A sore throat usually occurs as a result of an infection of the tonsils which often gives problems with swallowing.

Treatment

Apply the north-pole side of a magnet each side of the neck during the day.

Drink north-pole magnetised water three times a day.

Gargle with north-pole magnetised water twice a day.

THYMUS GLAND

The thymus gland is a small gland located behind the sternum and is responsible for keeping our immune system healthy so we can fight infections. Magnet therapy can help in keeping it functioning well.

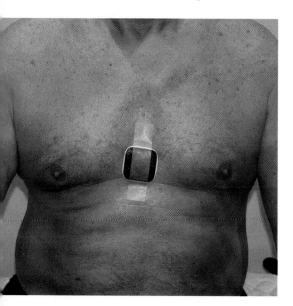

Treatment

Apply the north-pole side of a magnet or magnetic pad to the sternum for one hour twice a day.

Drink magnetised water three times a day.

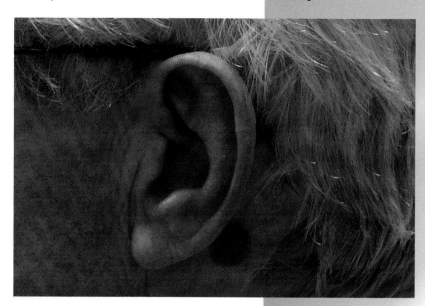

TINNITUS

Tinnitus is a continual buzzing, ringing or hissing in the ear, often caused by a loud noise or when the ear canals become blocked.

Treatment

General treatment with a magnetic pillow will help.

Apply the north side of a ½ inch neodymium magnet behind the ear during the day.

Below: tinnitus is a continual buzzing, ringing or hissing in the ear. Apply the north side of a ½ inch neodymium magnet behind the ear during the day.

Left: the thymus gland is a small gland located behind the sternum and is responsible for keeping our immune system healthy so we can fight infections. Apply the north-pole side of a magnet or magnetic pad to the sternum for one hour twice a day.

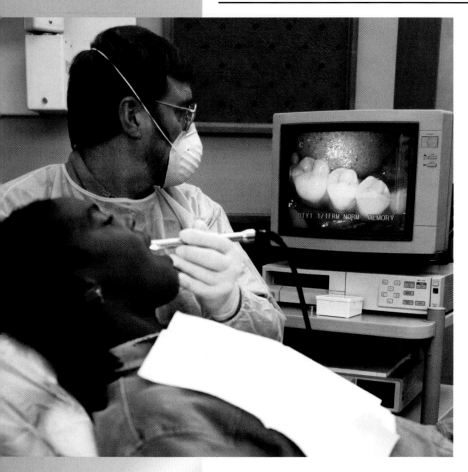

TRIGEMINAL NEURALGIA

Trigeminal neuralgia is a severe pain affecting one side of the face usually the cheek and jaw, normally of women in their forties and fifties. It can often occur after stress or exposure to cold or draughts.

Treatment

Sleep on a magnetic pillow

Apply the north side of a neodymium magnet to the affected area until pain subsides.

Use an electro-magnetic wand (a Magnessage) around the area for five minutes twice a day.

Drink magnetised water.

Above: magnet therapy can ease the pain of toothache until the dentist can be seen.

TOOTHACHE

A toothache is very unpleasant and normally only a visit to the dentist will stop the problem whether it be an infection or tooth trouble. Magnet therapy will, however, ease the pain until then.

Treatment

Apply the north-pole side of a magnet to the area of pain during the day.

Rinse the mouth with north-pole magnetised water twice a day.

Drink north-pole magnetised water.

VARICOSE VEINS

Varicose veins are dilated veins where the valves become weak and, as a result, the blood pools in the legs to form swollen veins.

Treatment

Wear magnetic insoles to help the blood circulation.

Tape the north-pole side of neodymium magnets close to the site for 15–20 minutes twice a day.

WARTS

Warts are small horny tumours on the skin caused by a virus infection. They are usually found on the hands or the feet where they are known as verrucas.

Treatment

Apply the north side of a neodymium magnet to the wart for several days.

Bathe the area in north-pole magnetised water twice a day.

Drink north-pole magnetised water twice a day.

WHIPLASH

Whiplash is a painful and restrictive condition of the neck normally caused by a car accident when the neck is wrenched in different directions.

Treatment

Sleep on a magnetic pillow.

Apply the north-pole side of two neodymium magnets to each side of the neck where the pain is felt during the day.

Massage with north-pole magnetised oil.

WRINKLES

Wrinkles are a fact of life, but can be reduced by the use of magnet therapy. A natural face lift and a younger look can also be achieved. As the blood circulation in the face increases so does the colour and muscle tone, giving a healthy young glow.

Treatment

Sleep on a magnetic pillow pad or mattress cover with magnets which are north-sided to the body.

Apply a magnetic eye mask or magnets over the problem areas on the forehead around the jawline and cheek bones for 30 minutes twice a day.

Massage the face with magnetised face creams.

Drink magnetised water twice a day.

REFERENCES

ACCREDITED THERAPISTS

Gloria Vergari MCMA
Norstar Biomagnetics
4th Street West
New Greenham Park
Newbury, RG19 6HN
Tel: 01635 586 650
email: gloria@norstarbiomagnetics.com
website: www.norstarbiomagnetics.com

Alan Cash MCMA
Priory House
Priory Road
West Kirby
Wirral CH48 7EU
tel: 0151 625 9355
email: cash.businesshouse@virgin.net

Lilias Curtin MCMA
30 Delvino Road
Fulham
London SW6 4AD
tel: 0207 731 4715
email: locurtin@aol.com

Valerie Dargonne MCMA BSYA (MT)
LCSP (Phys)
8 Sherbourne Road
Hove BN3 8BB
tel: 01273 421 077
mobile: 07803 269 418
email: valdargonne@yahoo.com

Jackie Hooper-Moore & Jenette
Atkins (Equestrian Specialists)
Old Station House
Axbridge
Somerset BS26 2AW
tel: 01934 733 325

Sue Kneebone
21 Bowden Hill
Laycock
Chippenham
tel: 01249 730 379

Alan Moyes MCMA
3 Fleece Cottages
Stanley Downton
Stroud GL10 3QU
tel: 01453 828 361
mobile: 07968 252 502

Celia Hitchen-Hilsley
Rose Cottage
Knutsford Road
Alderley Edge
Cheshire SK9 755
tel: 01565 873 753

Back 2
28 Wigmore Street
London WIH 9DF
tel: 0207 935 0351

For more up-to-date details of
accredited magnet therapists in your
area please call:

THE COMPLEMENTARY MEDICAL ASSOCIATION (CMA)

Tel: 0208 305 9571
Fax: 0208 305 4888
www.the-cma.org.uk

ACCREDITED COURSE INFORMATION

Valerie Dargonne MCMA, BSYA (MT),
LCSP (Phys)
88 Sherbourne Road
Hove BN3 8BB
tel: 01273 421 077
mobile: 07803 269 418

Coghill Research Labs
Ker Henez
Lower Race
Pontypool
Gwent NP4 5UF
tel: 01495 763 389

PRODUCTS WE LIKE

Norstar Biomagnetics
(Helpline available)
High quality theraputic products
Wraps and disks
The Magnessage
Sleep systems
tel: 01635 568 650
fax: 01635 568 651
email: info@norstarbiomagnetics.com
website: www.norstarbiomagnetics.com

Magnotec
Magnetic device
tel: 0208 670 5883
fax: 0208 766 6616

Homedics UK Limited
Economic magnetic products
Wraps etc.
19 Branksome Avenue
Prestwich
Manchester M25 1AG

INDEX